Minimally Invasive Techniques/Structural Heart Disease

Edited By

Dr. Peter M. Schofield
Papworth Hospital
UK

Minimally Invasive Techniques for the Treatment of Patients with Structural Heart Disease

Editor: Peter M. Schofield

eISBN: 978-1-60805-119-9

ISBN: 978-1-60805-684-2

© 2011, Bentham eBooks imprint.

Published by Bentham Science Publishers – Sharjah, UAE. All Rights Reserved.

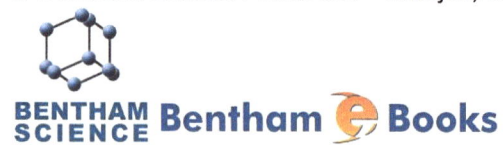

BENTHAM SCIENCE Bentham e Books

CONTENTS

FOREWORD

Interventional cardiology has evolved on a rapid and broad front in the last 20 years. Coronary intervention is now established with well designed and functional equipment. Some aspects of non-coronary intervention are long standing such as balloon valvuloplasty on aortic, pulmonary and mitral valves and the technology and techniques are mature in these small areas. Defect closure has developed and the treatment has become the first choice for such patients. However valve disease is a major cause of morbidity and mortality in our aging population and becoming a major health problem. The enclosed work considers the non surgical approaches that are available. Percutaneous aortic and mitral valve interventions are likely to be the future of the management of valve disease, as are electronic books.

Dr. Len Shapiro
Papworth Hospital
UK

PREFACE

Historically, patients with advanced structural heart disease have required major surgery to correct the defect. This includes for example, patients with atrial septal defect, aortic valve disease and mitral valve disease. In recent years there have been major advances in the treatment of patients with structural heart disease using minimally invasive, percutaneous treatments. This field continues to evolve quite quickly.

This e-book outlines the current situation in respect of the minimally invasive treatment of a wide range of structural cardiac defects. As the technology continues to develop, we aim to modify the book to keep-up-to date with new developments.

In each chapter we aim to cover details of the structural defect in question and outline the various technologies available for treating the condition. We include the indications for the procedure as well as providing details of the procedure itself. Finally, we present the outcomes of the use of the devices.

Chapter 1 PFO Closure

The clinical presentation of patients with a patent foramen ovale is described. The imaging techniques used for this condition are discussed. An important area is the indications for percutaneous closure of PFO, and also selecting patients who do not need to have a closure device. The outcomes of clinical trials in this field are presented which will guide patient selection.

Chapter 2 Atrial Septal Defect

This chapter deals with the classification of the different types of atrial septal defect. It outlines the presenting symptoms of patients with this condition, and also outlines the investigations required for patient management, with the typical findings. It presents the pros and cons of percutaneous closure of an atrial septal defect with the alternative option of surgical closure. The different types of device available for ASD closure are described and discussed in detail. The outcomes of percutaneous closure are also described.

Chapter 3 Transcutaneous Aortic Valve Implantation

The different types of device available for transcutaneous aortic valve implantation are described. The pros and cons of the different devices are discussed. The current indications for transcutaneous aortic valve implantation are outlined. The current situation regarding this technology is presented, and compared with the outcomes of open heart surgery in the high risk population. The outcomes of TAVI are also described and potential future developments in this area are discussed.

Chapter 4 Balloon Valvuloplasty

The role of balloon valvuloplasty in patients who have aortic stenosis (when balloon valvuloplasty may be used prior to transcutaneous aortic valve implantation), mitral stenosis, pulmonary stenosis or tricuspid stenosis are discussed. The specific indications for balloon valvuloplasty in patients with these various structural abnormalities are described. The outcomes of balloon valvuloplasty in these different patient populations are presented. The technique of balloon valvuloplasty in these various conditions is also outlined in detail.

Chapter 5 Mitral Regurgitation – Leaflet Technologies

The various types of device which involve treating the mitral valve leaflets are described. The selection of patients for treatment using these technologies are presented in detail. The pros and cons of these devices are described, together with a comparison with mitral valve repair using a surgical approach. The outcomes following treatment by percutaneous technologies are described, as are potential future developments in this area.

Chapter 6 Mitral Regurgitation – "Coronary Sinus" Technologies

The different types of device available using a coronary sinus approach are described. Their mechanism of action is also outlined. The selection of patients for treatment using this technology is discussed, together with the various investigations which the patients require prior to treatment. The outcomes of treating patients with these devices are presented, and potential future developments in this area are discussed.

Chapter 7 – Left Atrial Appendage Occlusion Devices

The technologies available are described, together with the techniques for their implantation. An important area is the selection of patients for these devices. The outcomes of treatment with these devices is described, and potential future developments in this area are discussed.

In summary, therefore the book is clinically orientated, and provides a comprehensive and up to date description of the use of many devices in clinical practice. Since the area is rapidly evolving, the book needs to be revised at fairly frequent intervals.

Dr. Peter M. Schofield
Papworth Hospital
UK

List of Contributors

David Begley

Papworth Hospital, Cambridge, UK

Patrick Calvert

Papworth Hospital, Cambridge, UK

Cameron Densem Papworth

Hospital, Cambridge, UK

David Hildick-Smith Brighton

University Hospital, UK

Stephen Hoole

Papworth Hospital, Cambridge, UK

Michael O'Sullivan Papworth

Hospital, Cambridge, UK

Liam Mccormick Papworth

Hospital, Cambridge, UK

Daniel Obaid

Papworth Hospital, Cambridge, UK

Rebecca Schofield

Peterborough District Hospital, Cambridge, UK

CHAPTER 1

Percutaneous Closure of Patent Foramen Ovale (PFO)

Stephen Hoole[*]

Papworth Hospital. Cambridge, UK

Abstract: Patent foramen ovale (PFO) is a common anatomical finding in a quarter of the general population and under certain conditions may shunt clot, deoxygenated blood or gas bubbles right-to-left across the atrial septum to cause cryptogenic stroke, platypnoea orthodeoxia or decompression illness respectively. PFO has also been linked to migraine with aura. Treatment by percutaneous closure as a day case is technically feasible and has been aided by the recent development of intracardiac and 3D transoesophageal imaging, as well as improvements in device technology. The results from several large randomised controlled trials designed to assess superiority of PFO closure above medical therapy alone for cryptogenic stroke are eagerly awaited.

ANATOMY AND PHYSIOLOGY

The foramen ovale is a flap valve remnant of foetal circulation, formed antero-superiorly by the septum secundum and infero-posteriorly by the septum primum. In normal foetal circulation oxygenated venous blood from the placenta travels up the inferior vena cava (IVC) and is directed across the foramen ovale to the left atrium and from there the systemic circulation, bypassing the lungs. Following the new-born's first breath, lung expansion causes the right atrial pressure to diminish below the left atrial pressure and the septum primum is opposed onto the septum secundum. This eventually seals by prostaglandin E1 dependent septal fusion, occurring within the first year of life in 65-80% of individuals to form the fossa ovalis.

Anatomical variants within the atria may contribute to failure of the atrial septum to seal (Fig. **1A** and **B**). A prominent Eustacian valve from the inferior vena cava increases blood flow towards the foramen ovale, whilst a mobile atrial septal aneurysm (ASA) can pull the flap open with every heart beat. The combination of septal separation and increased flow prevents septal adherence and fusion.

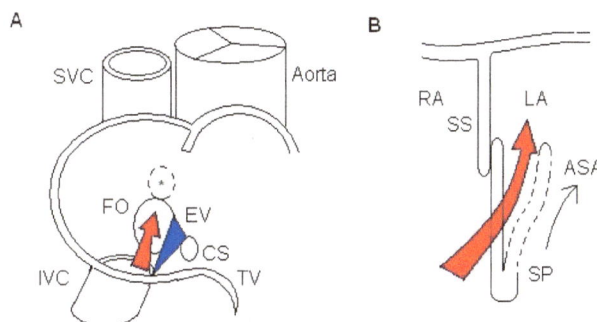

Figure 1A: Schematic diagram of the atrial septum viewed from the right atrium (RA). Blood is directed towards the foramen ovale (FO) by the Eustacian valve (EV - blue), particularly when this ridge is prominent. Blood can then flow into the left atrium (LA) *via* the left atrial PFO orifice (*). B: Perpendicular section through the atrial septum demonstrating that right-to-left shunting is further encouraged when there is a large atrial septal aneurysm (ASA) affecting the septum primum (SP) or secundum (SS).

EPIDEMIOLOGY

The prevalence in the general population of probe patent foramen ovale ranges from 15-25% in autopsy studies. In one such registry that studied 965 normal hearts, the overall incidence was 27.3% [1] Interestingly the prevalence diminished with increasing age (1st-3rd decade: 34.3%, 4th-8th decade: 25.4%, 9th-10th decade: 20.2%) perhaps hinting

---

*****Address correspondence to Stephen Hoole:** Papworth Hospital. Cambridge, UK; E-mail: stevieh@doctors.org.uk

of a survival disadvantage in individuals with a PFO. The average size of the PFO also increased with age (1st decade: 3.4mm vs. 10th decade: 5.8mm). The prevalence of PFO from clinical registries based on echocardiographic detection is in broad agreement with autopsy registry data (although variability exists due to different detection rates with transthoracic and transoesophageal echocardiography). However, in patients with a prior history of cerebral embolus or migraine the prevalence can rise to 40-50% [2,3].

ASSOCIATIONS AND COMPLICATIONS

Right-to-left Shunt

The PFO accounts for approximately 95% of all right-to-left shunts in humans. The remainder are mainly due to pulmonary arteriovenous fistulas (4%) or atrial septal defects (1%). Right-to-left shunting *via* the PFO can rarely cause *Platypnoea Orthodeoxia Syndrome*. Deoxygenated venous blood from the inferior vena cava is shunted from right atrium to left atrium *via* the PFO on standing, despite normal right heart pressures. This leads to cyanosis and breathlessness, which is relieved in the recumbent position. Theories abound as to why this occurs, including compression of the right atrium during upright posture, decreased right ventricular compliance and an unfavourable orientation of the inferior vena cava to the atrial septum.

Paradoxical Embolism

When shunting right to left, a PFO can enable clot that has developed in the systemic veins or in the foramen tunnel itself to access the left heart and systemic circulation to cause a *paradoxical embolism*. Under normal physiological conditions the left atrial pressure (LAP) is greater than right atrial pressure (RAP) and the flap of the septum primum occludes the foramen ovale. However, when there is a transient increase in RAP (as occurs during a sneeze, cough and the release phase of a Valsalva manoeuvre) right to left shunting may occur at the level of the atrium, facilitating the translocation of clot.

Similarly, increased right heart pressures secondary to previous pulmonary emboli can increase the risk of subsequent paradoxical embolism. In a study of patients with clinically apparent pulmonary embolism, the mere presence of a PFO increased mortality from 14% to 33% and systemic embolism from 2% to 28% (p<0.02) [4] A causal link between PFO and paradoxical embolism is further strengthened by case reports of threatened paradoxical embolism detected by transoesophageal echocardiography - organised thrombus from a saphenous vein cast can sometimes be demonstrated lodged within the PFO "en route" to the systemic circulation (Fig. **2**).

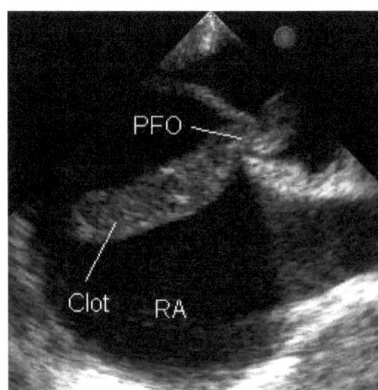

Figure 2: Threatened paradoxical embolism shown on TOE.

Paradoxical emboli are rare in children and young adults but increase in frequency with age, particularly after 50 years of age. Most thrombi emerge from the inferior vena cava and are encouraged to cross a PFO if a large Eustacian valve (increasing flow towards the PFO) or atrial septal aneurysm (pulling the PFO open) are both present. One or both of these features are present in 2-4% of the population. The coexistence of an ASA with a PFO increases the risk of embolic stroke (PFO alone HR 0.86 (0.31-2.36), p=0.77 vs. PFO and ASA HR 4.97 (1.47-11.84), p=0.007) [5]. Cryptogenic stroke is a common diagnosis, accounting for approximately 40% of all ischaemic strokes [6]. Paradoxical embolism can also cause myocardial, eye, and visceral infarction as well as arterial limb embolism.

Decompression Illness

This occurs when dissolved nitrogen or helium in the blood comes out solution during rapid depressurisation, most commonly during rapid ascent from a long, deep dive. Micro-bubbles preferentially form in venous blood and are filtered by the lungs. However, in the presence of a PFO micro-bubbles can shunt from right-to-left and cause arterial gas embolism in tissues, sometimes with catastrophic consequences. A study has revealed that the incidence of PFO in divers with previous decompression illness was 77% compared with 27% of control group divers [7]. Larger PFO defects were particularly associated with the cutaneous and neourological (spinal) decompression illness.

Migraine

There is a presumed causal association between PFO and classical migraine *with aura*, although the underlying aetiology is poorly understood. Retrospective data have shown that migraine headache with aura is associated with large PFO that spontaneously shunt right-to-left [8]. It is postulated that vasoactive substances and microemboli that are normally filtered by the lungs, pass into and irritate the cerebral circulation [9].

DIAGNOSTIC IMAGING

Non-invasive

TTE

Transthoracic echo alone does not have adequate sensitivity to rule-out the diagnosis of PFO, although when combined with a bubble study the sensitivity of the test is improved.

Bubble Study

A transthoracic echo with bubble study can be used to assess the presence and size (number of bubbles) of a right-to-left shunt, but is highly dependent on the patient and the operator performing the study. A bubble study is positive if >5 micro-bubbles are observed in the left atrium within 3 beats of right atrial opacification. This is termed spontaneous if it occurs without a Valsalva. If micro-bubbles are seen after 5 beats then pulmonary arteriovenous fistula may be present. A large number of micro-bubbles (>30) in the left atrium indicates a large right-to-left shunt (**Movie 1**).

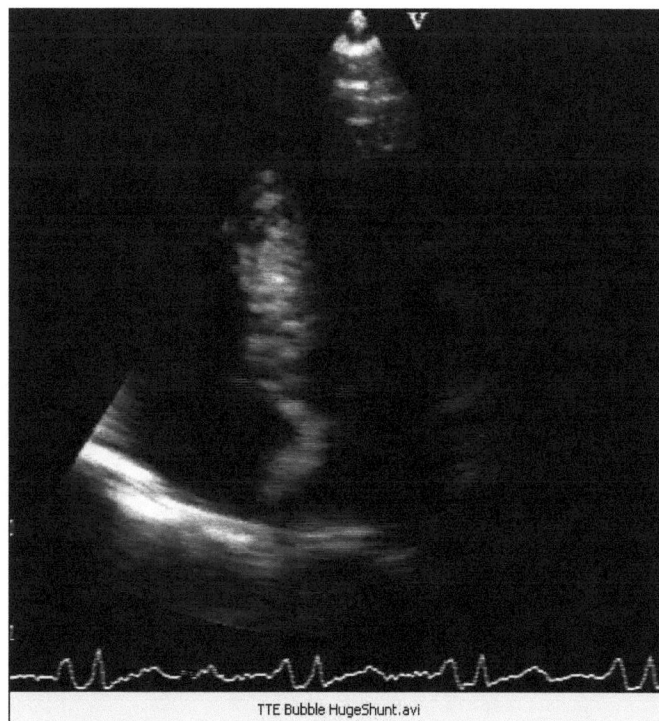

TTE Bubble HugeShunt.avi

Movie 1: TTE (A4C view) during a positive bubble study demonstrating a large right-to-left shunt across a PFO.

Tips and Tricks

Quality control on the recorded bubble study should be performed to improve diagnostic accuracy. In particular, the operator should ensure that the right atrium was fully opacified with micro-bubbles. This is achieved by vigorous mixing of 1mL venous blood with 9 mL saline and air between 2 x 10mL Luer lock syringes connected to a 3-way tap. This should be injected into a large vein followed by a large saline flush. If a Valsalva manoeuvre is performed to provoke a right-to-left shunt, it should be practised by the patient (instructing the patient to attempt to blow the stopper out of a syringe is often helpful) and the technician must ensure that the atria remain in the field of view during the release phase. An atrial septal bulged from the right-to-left confirms a successful Valsalva release. Sniffing can also precipitate micro-bubble right-to-left shunting, as can injections *via* a femoral vein, as the inferior vena cava preferentially delivers the micro-bubbles directly onto the enface atrial septum.

Invasive

TOE

Pre-procedural and/or intra-operative assessment of the PFO and surrounding structures can be achieved with transoesophageal echocardiography (TOE). In particular, the increased resolution enables more detailed assessment of PFO anatomy (**Movie 2**: PFO and ASA) and flow with colour-flow Doppler (**Movie 3**: PFO colour flow Doppler), detection of small right-to-left shunts with bubble study, and confirmation that additional potential shunts (ASD, fenestrations and anomalous pulmonary veins) are absent. Intra-operative TOE also offers other advantages including confirmation that the left atrial appendage is empty, information on the PFO retraction on the wire, device conformation, position and alignment prior to release (**Movie 4**), device impingement on surrounding structures and the prompt detection of complications, such as tamponade. The recent development of real-time 3D transoesophageal echocardiography has further increased the utility of this imaging modality (**Movies 5-7**).

However, TOE is uncomfortable for the patient with risks of aspiration and oesophageal trauma and often necessitates general anaesthetic if used intraoperatively.

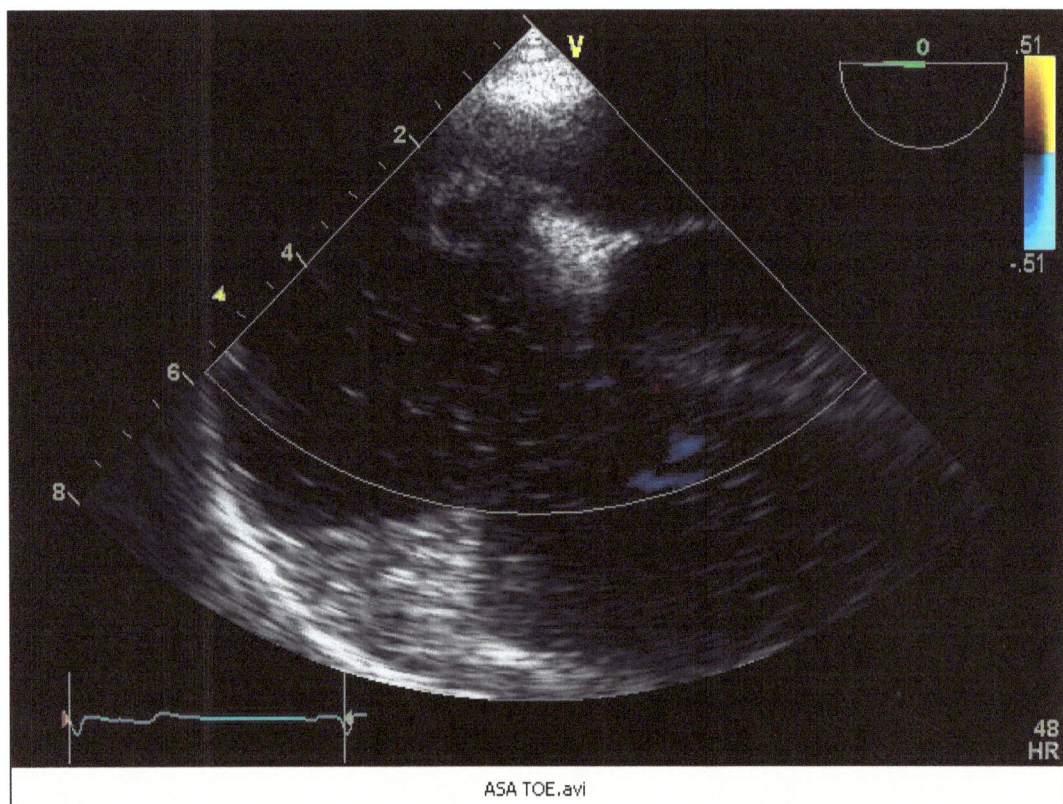

Movie 2: TOE demonstrating an atrial septal aneurysm.

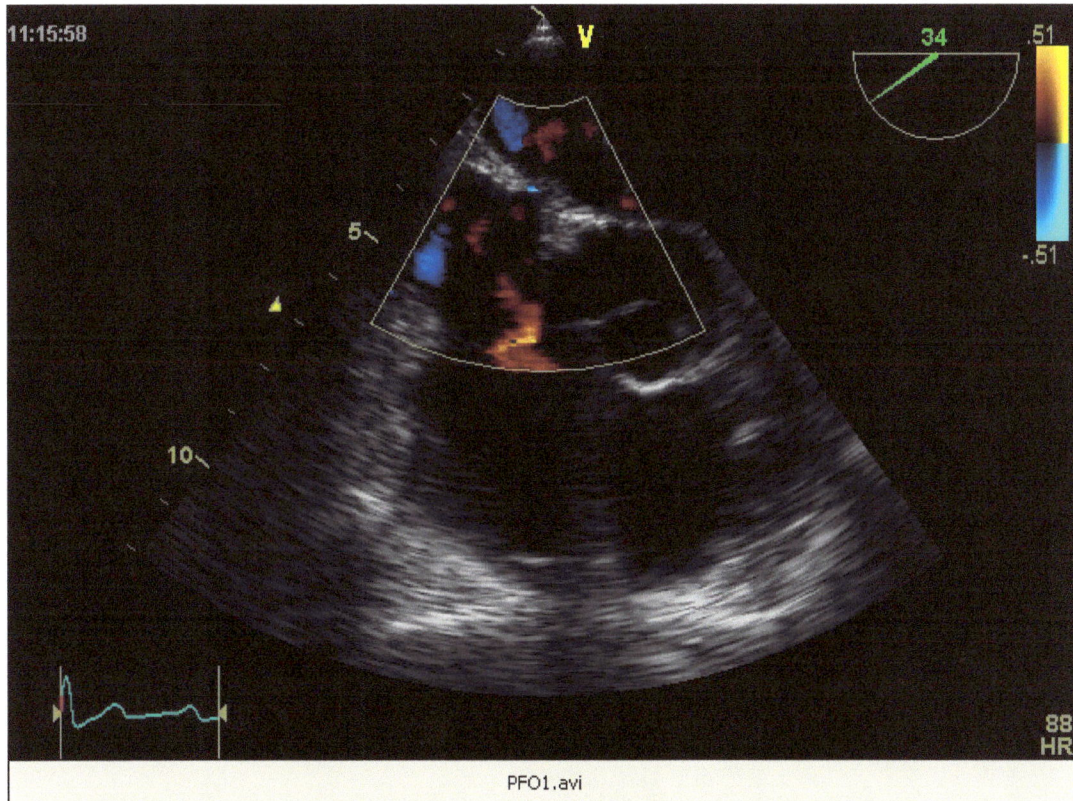

Movie 3: TOE with colour flow Doppler demonstrating flow within the PFO.

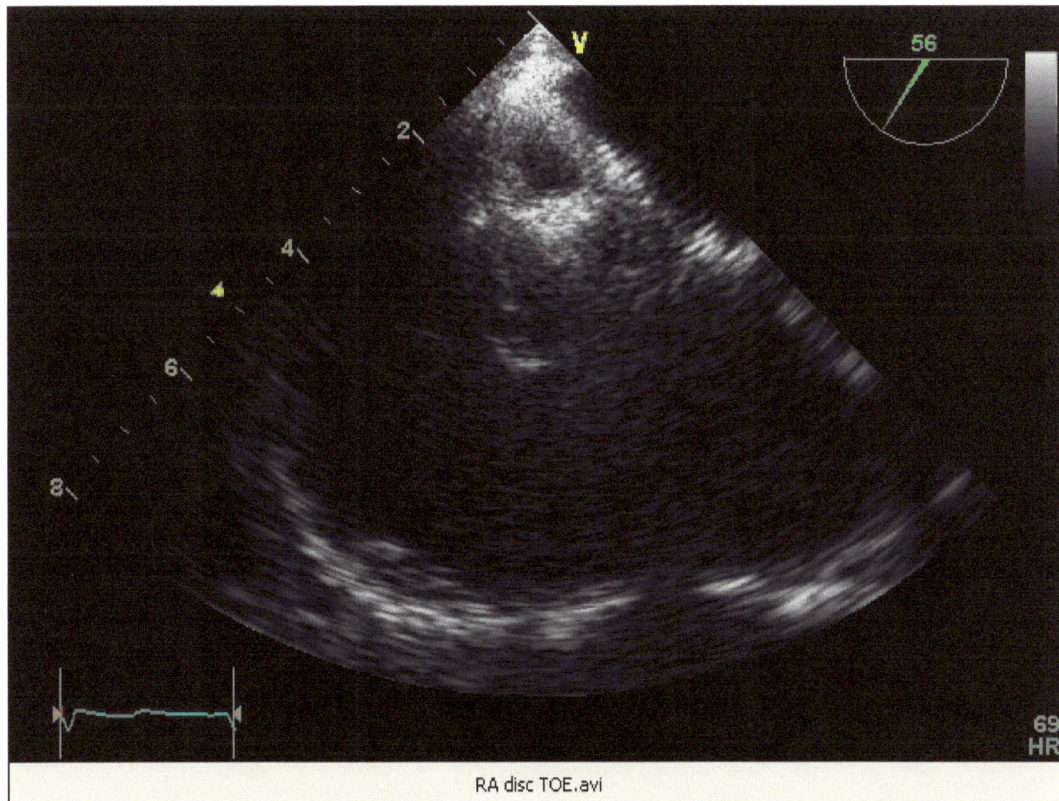

Movie 4: TOE of an Amplatzer PFO Occluder with the RA disc pulled of the septum due to tension from the delivery cable.

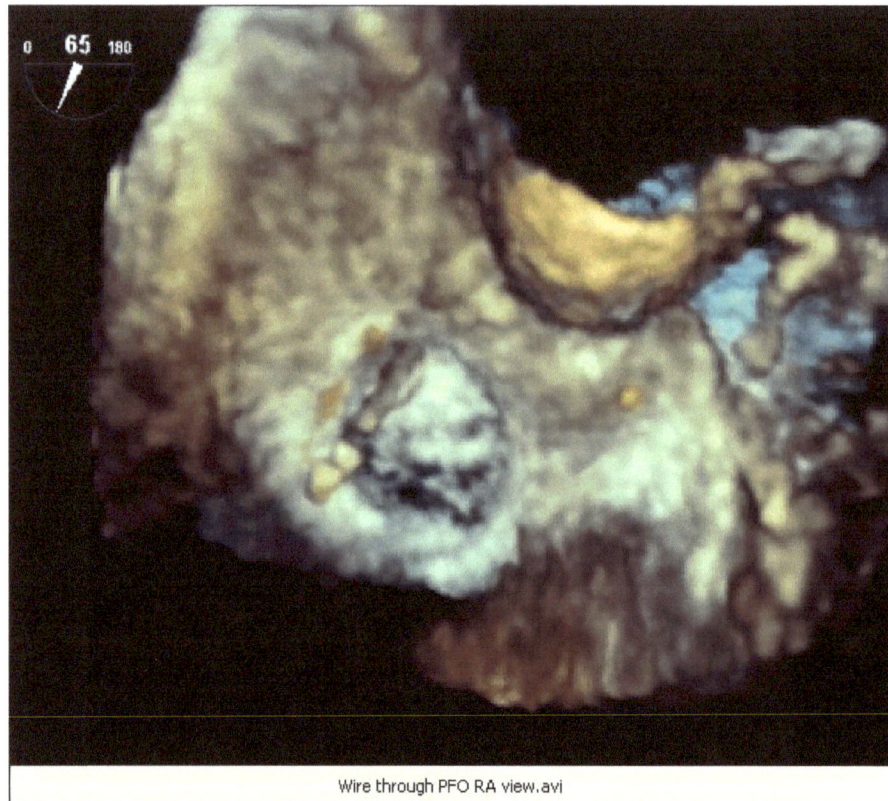

Movie 5: 3D TOE (right atrial view) demonstrating a wire across the PFO.

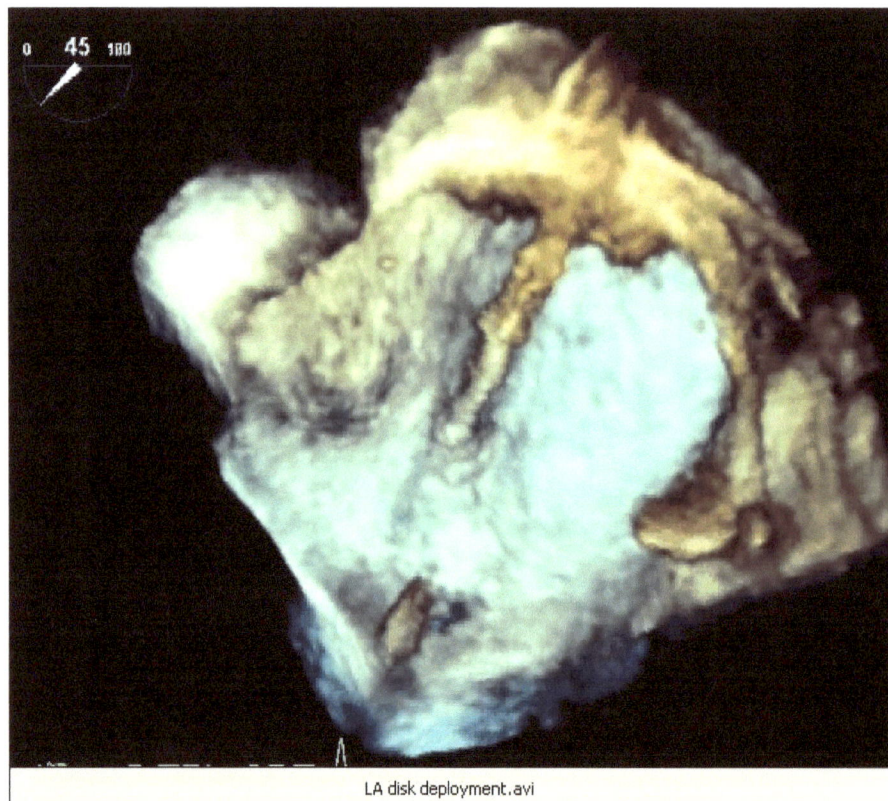

Movie 6: 3D TOE (left atrial view) showing left atrial disc deployment of a BioSTAR device.

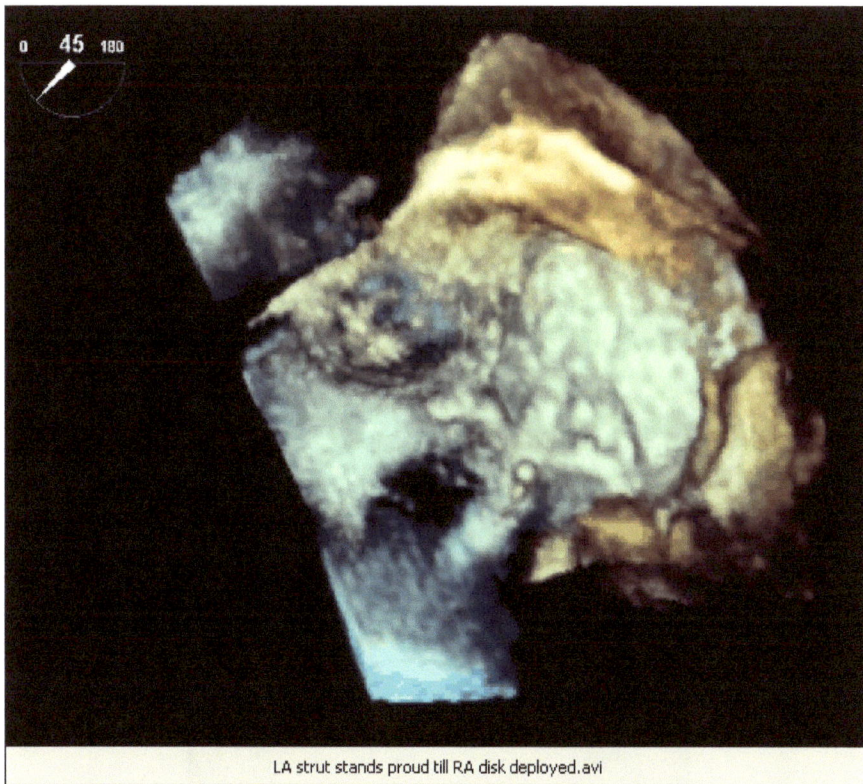

LA strut stands proud till RA disk deployed.avi

Movie 7: 3D TOE (left atrial view) showing release of the right atrial disc of a BioSTAR device with conformational change of the whole device due to reduced tension.

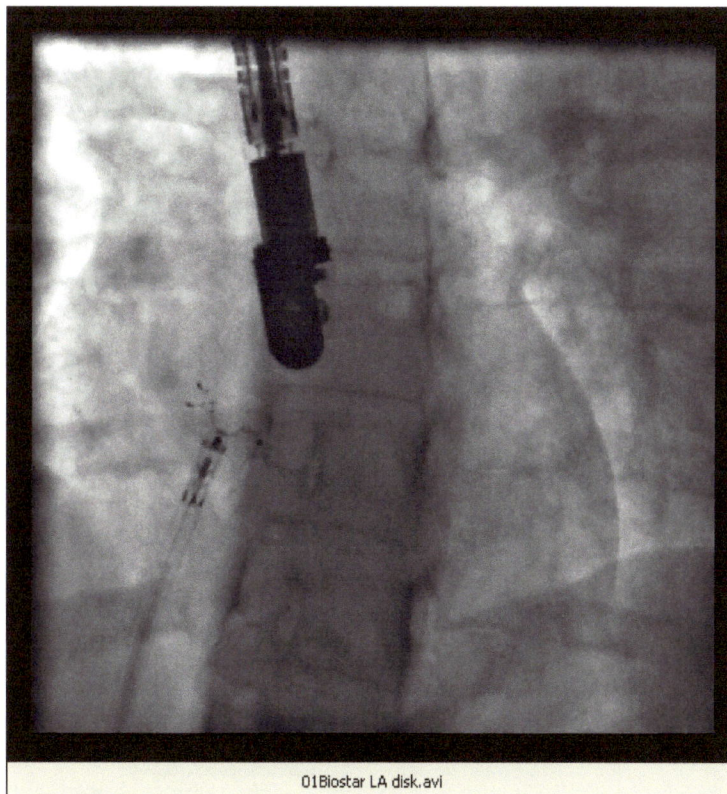

01Biostar LA disk.avi

Movie 8: LAO view of deployment of the left atrial disc of a BioSTAR device.

ICE

Similar high quality imaging of the atrial septum and PFO can be achieved from intra-cardiac echocardiography (ICE) using the AcuNAV™ system *via* an 8F venous sheath. The advantage of this is that the procedure can be performed without general anaesthetic as a day case. However, there are cost implications in using the single use ICE probe, and doubling of the risk of venous access complications. In addition, as there is no or minimal left-to-right shunting with PFO, the right atrium is often of normal, small dimensions, which can limit the views of the PFO and surrounding structures.

Contrast Fluoroscopy

Visualisation of the PFO by contrast injection can often be performed during the closure procedure, *via* the side-arm of the introducer sheath. Optimal views of the PFO are achieved from 20° right anterior oblique with 20° cranial tilt or 20-40° left anterior oblique with 10° caudal tilt. Peri-procedural fluoroscopy aides PFO closure device implantation (**Movies 4 -6**) and may be used as the only intra-procedural imaging modality if the PFO anatomy is straight forward (small PFO with a short tunnel and no ASA) [10].

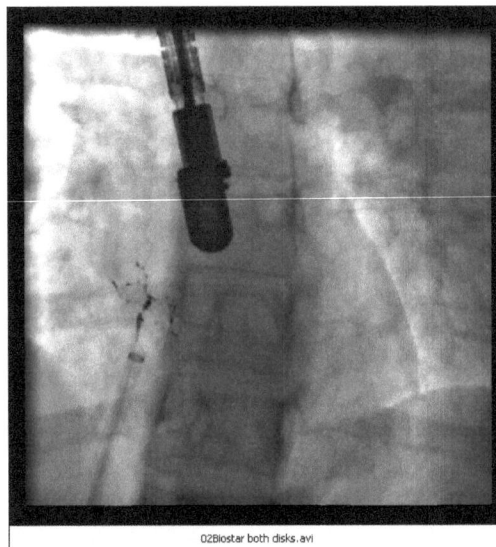

Movie 9: LAO view of the right atrial disc of a BioSTAR device.

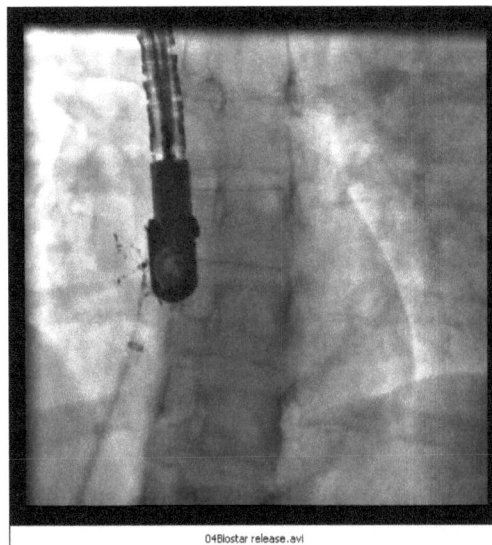

Movie 10: LAO view of BioSTAR device release.

TREATMENT

Cryptogenic Stroke

Medical

Current guidelines on the treatment of patients with PFO and cerebral events concentrate on conservative therapeutic options. Comparison of warfarin vs. aspirin thromboprophylaxis in patients with PFO and cryptogenic stroke was studied in the warfarin-aspirin recurrent stroke study [11]. Ischaemic stroke recurrence or death rate was equivalent between treatment strategies (2 year event rates: warfarin 9.5% vs. aspirin 17.9%, p=0.28). Warfarin is recommended for patients with PFO, cryptogenic stroke and coexistent deep vein thrombosis, coagulation disorder and/or an atrial septal aneurysm. Otherwise aspirin provides adequate stroke thromboprophylaxis.

Surgical Closure

This is rarely indicated as an isolated procedure, although may be performed during surgery for another reason with good results [12].

Percutaneous Closure

There are no large randomised clinical trials comparing treatment options for the main indication for PFO closure – cryptogenic stroke. However, there are several large trials currently evaluating the role of percutaneous closure of PFO for this condition (Table 1). Retrospective and small non-randomised prospective studies have shown comparable recurrent stroke rates (5-10% over 2 years follow-up) for device closure with medical treatment [13-15]. Possible explanations of treatment parity include clot formation on the device and/or incomplete closure of the PFO.

Table 1: Clinical trials of PFO Closure for Cryptogenic Stroke

Trial	Device	Start	Finance	Target n	Status	Publication	www.clinicaltrials.gov
PC	Amplatzer PFO	2000	AGA Medical	450	Finished enrolment	2011	NCT00166257
Closure-1	STARFlex	2003	NMT Medical	1600	Finished enrolment	2011	NCT00201461
RESPECT	Amplatzer PFO	2004	AGA Medical	900	Enrolling	2013	N/A
CLOSE	Any	2007	Public	900	Enrolling	2014	NCT00562289
REDUCE	HELEX	2008	WL Gore	664	Enrolling	2016	NCT00738894

PC: PFO and cryptogenic embolism; Closure-1: Evaluation of the STARFlex septal closure system with patients with a stroke or transient ischaemic attack caused by the possible passage of a clot of unknown origin through a PFO; RESPECT: Randomised evaluation of recurrent stroke comparing PFO closure and established current standard of care treatment; CLOSE: PFO closure and anticoagulants versus antiplatelet therapy to prevent stroke recurrence; REDUCE: HELEX septal occluder for PFO closure in stroke patients.

Percutaneous PFO closure is currently only recommended in patients with recurrent cryptogenic stroke despite warfarin therapy and those patients with contraindications to anticoagulation. Percutaneous closure is contraindicated in patients with evidence of thrombus in the left atrium. Patients with nickel allergy may still be closed with devices that are not made of nitinol.

Decompression illness

Professional divers and caisson workers are often offered percutaneous closure to prevent paradoxical gas embolism and to enable them to return to employment. However, there are no trial data to support PFO closure for this indication.

Migraine

Although anecdotal evidence exist that migraine headache symptoms improve after PFO closure [16,17], there are no randomised controlled trials that have unequivocally shown a benefit of PFO closure to reduce the frequency of migraine headache. Despite early encouraging results from an interim analysis, the controversial MIST (Migraine

Intervention with STARFlex Technology) trial did not demonstrate headache cessation or even a reduction in the frequency of headache with aura, following PFO closure [18]. PFO closure for migraine headache with aura is not currently recommended.

PERCUTANEOUS PFO CLOSURE

Pre-procedural Preparation

Cryptogenic stroke due to PFO is a diagnosis of exclusion and therefore other potential causes of stoke should be investigated prior to PFO closure. These include: head and neck vessel imaging with MRA, CT or ultrasonography, detailed echocardiography to exclude other structural heart disease (e.g. ASD and anomalous pulmonary venous drainage), a thrombophilia screen (Protein C and S, antithrombin, factor V Leiden, anticardiolipin antibody) and an ECG to screen for atrial fibrillation.

If patients are anticoagulated with warfarin this should be replaced with aspirin 2-5 days prior to procedure to minimise peri-procedural bleeding complications. Pre-procedural antibiotic prophylaxis is recommended.

Procedure

The first transcatheter closure of a PFO with an umbrella device was performed by Lock and colleagues in 1987 [19]. The simplest and most widely used device used today to close PFO is the Amplatzer PFO Occluder. Implantation of this device is summarised below, although many of the steps are common to all devices.

Access:

- Femoral venous sheath 9F
- Intravenous heparin 70-100iu/kg
- Cross the PFO with 6F Multipurpose or Judkins right 4 diagnostic catheter and a 0.035" exchange length wire
- Leave the 0.035" wire in the left upper pulmonary vein
- Remove the catheter and 9F sheath

Device preparation:

- Select the smallest diameter device that will successfully close the PFO
- Soak in warm saline
- Attach to delivery cable by clockwise cable rotation
- Retract into loading catheter under water and de-air with repeated flushing with a saline filled Luer lock syringe *via* the O-ring

Implantation:

- After flushing the delivery sheath and introducer pass both over the wire into mid LA
- Remove the introducer and 0.035" wire and de-air under water
- Engage the loading catheter under water and push the cable and device into the delivery sheath
- Push the LA disc out of the distal delivery sheath into the mid LA
- Pull delivery sheath and cable back *together* until resistance (may confirm seal with contrast injection or echo)
- Pull back delivery sheath to deploy the RA disc
- Test device stability (optional in PFO) with the "Minnesota wiggle"

- Release device with anti-clockwise turns on the cable and pull cable into delivery sheath

- Exchange the delivery sheath for a 12F venous sheath to achieve haemostasis

Tips and Tricks

Avoiding Air

This can be achieved by scrupulous de-airing during every stage of the procedure. We prepare the device completely submerged in a water bath and insure that all the Luer locks on the loading catheter are wet to guarantee air-tight seals. In addition, the delivery sheath is de-aired by passive bleed back and the device loaded under water *below* the level of the left atrium.

Avoiding Perforation

The Amplatzer PFO Occluder can usually be successfully implanted without using the Amplatzer Super-stiff wire, which can readily perforate the thin walled left atrial appendage. A 0.035" J-tiped exchange length wire usually provides adequate support. Pulling the delivery cable into the sheath after device release also minimises the risk of perforation.

Ensuring Successful Device Release

A half turn anticlockwise after locking the device onto the delivery cable ensures that it will easily release after successful implantation. Avoid further turns on the cable during implantation.

Balloon Sizing

This is advocated particularly if the tunnel of the PFO is long, to assess tunnel morphology and degree of flap retraction prior to deciding on closure strategy (Fig. **3**). However, routine balloon sizing is not necessary as most PFO are small (4-6mm) short tunnels that stretch minimally.

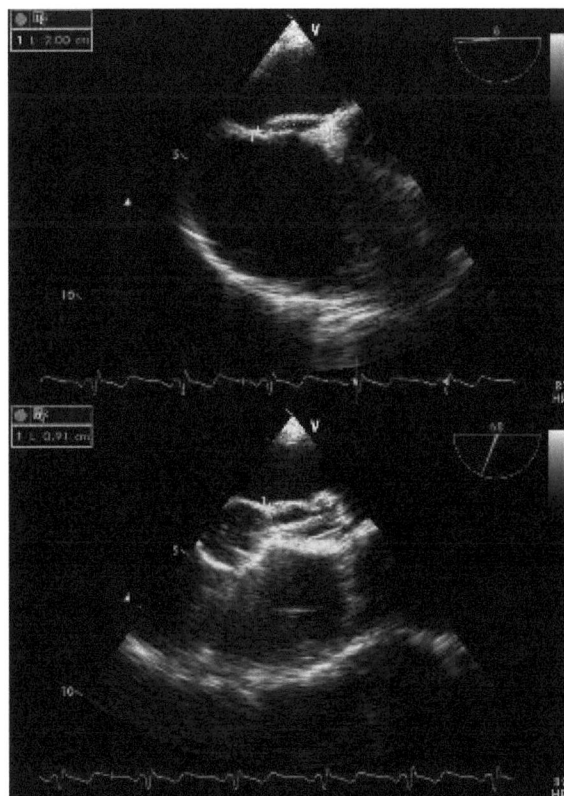

Figure 3: Balloon sizing.

Types of Closure Device

Percutaneous PFO closure devices essentially share similar structural attributes (Fig. **4** Table **2**). They have a wire frame (often made of the memory metal nitinol) with one or two patches or umbrella shaped discs connected to a waist. Newer generation devices minimise material in the left atrium that could act as a nidus for thrombus formation and have bioabsorbable components to facilitate endothelialisation and healing. To this end, totally bioabsorbable devices, the PFO stitch and radiofrequency ablation technology are under development with the aim of sealing the PFO without leaving any trace in the atrial septum.

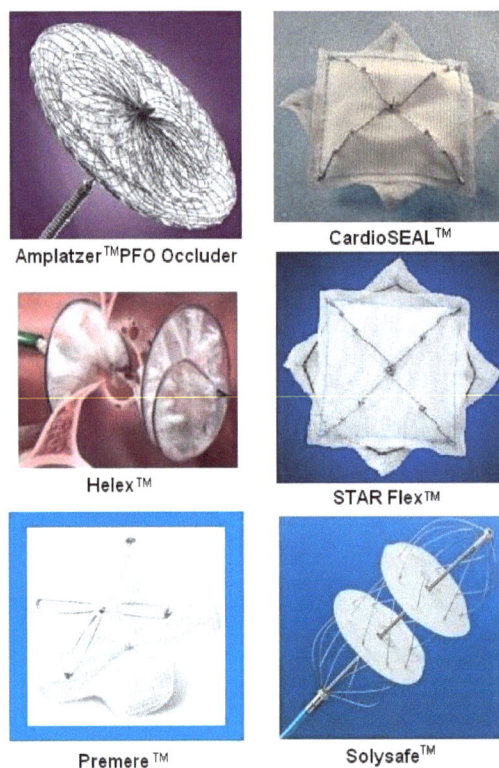

Figure 4: Commonly used closure devices.

Table 2: Closure device product characteristics.

Device	Frame	Patch/ Disc	Defect Size (Device Sizes)	Delivery Sheath
Amplatzer™ PFO Occluder	Nitinol	Polyester	9 – 17.5mm (18, 25, 30, 35mm)	8-9F
STARFlex™	MP35N	Polyester	13.5 – 22mm (23, 28, 33, 38mm)	10F (12F – 38mm)
BioSTAR™	Nitinol	Collagen matrix	n/a (23, 28 and 33mm)	11F
HELEX™	Nitinol	ePTFE	7.5 – 17.5mm (15, 20, 25, 30, 35mm)	10F
Premere™	Nitinol	Polyester	7.5 - 15mm (15, 20, 25mm)	11F
Solysafe™	Phynox	Polyester	4 – 30 mm (Type 15, 20, 25, 30, 35)	10F (12F - 30 /35)

Matching Closure Device to the Anatomy

Anatomical variations that are present in patients with PFO should be taken into account when selecting the appropriate type of PFO closure device.

PFO and ASA

The atrial septum is often highly mobile with redundant tissue in ASA, causing the PFO to gape open, potentially leading to device instability. A larger, bulkier closure devices e.g. Amplatzer PFO Occluder is indicated to prevent device embolization.

Fixed long PFO Tunnel

The septum primum and secundum cannot be easily opposed to seal the PFO with the flimsier devices and the long tunnel can cause the patches to fold inwards into the tunnel, resulting in device embolization. The Premere PFO Occluder has a variable length tether and a right atrial patch and left atrial anchor that can independently orientate to the left and right atrial septum walls to achieve a good seal. Alternative approaches include implantation of a larger bulkier device e.g. Amplatzer PFO Occluder, or performing a trans-septal puncture before implanting the closure device to achieve left and right atrial disc alignment.

Flap retraction and Thick Atrial Septum

In this scenario, infero-posterior retraction of the septum primum can occur when the wire is across the PFO, essentially converting the PFO into an ASD (or PFD – patent foramen defect) with corrugation of bulky septal tissue. This, in addition to thick atrial septal tissue can prevent the atrial discs of the device from lying flat and sealing the PFO. The flimsier devices may then stent the PFO open and exacerbate the shunt.

Complications

Successful device implantation occurs in approximately 98% of cases although complications secondary to device implantation are recognised (Table **3**).

Table 3: Complications of percutaneous PFO closure

Early	Incidence
Puncture site haematoma / vascular injury	2-4%
AF / Atrial tachycardia	1-2%
ST elevation	1.4-3.9%
TIA	0.3-0.8%
Pericardial Effusion / Tamponade	0.4-1.8%
Device embolism	<1%
Late	
Erosion	<0.1%
Thrombus	0-6.6%
Chest pain	1%
New onset migraine	1%

Early Complications

Atrial arrhythmias during the procedure are not uncommon but are usually transient and rarely require long term treatment. Transient ST elevation, particularly in the inferior ECG leads is also observed and is invariably due to air embolism. When the patient is supine, bubbles "float" to the anterior placed right coronary sinus. This usually settles with high flow oxygen, although occasionally coronary intervention is necessary.

Late Complications

Thrombus formation on the device is particularly associated with coexistent atrial fibrillation and/or atrial septal aneurysms. New onset migraine has been linked with platelet aggregation and micro-emboli liberated from the device. This can be treated with clopidogrel. Chest pain and malaise has been linked to nickel allergy but usually settles with non-steroidal anti-inflammatory treatment, although sometimes steroids are required.

Post Procedure

Most correctly implanted devices will endothelialise within 12 weeks and complete closure (confirmed by 6-month follow-up bubble study) is reported in 51-98% of cases. Therefore patients should continue their pre-procedural anticoagulation until PFO sealing has been confirmed. Patients on warfarin may gain additional benefit from anti-platelet therapy. We recommend 6 months treatment of aspirin and/or clopidogrel following PFO closure in treatment naïve patients.

REFERENCES

[1]   Hagen PT, Scholtz DG, Edwards WD *et al.* Incidence and size of patent foramen ovale during the first ten decades of life: an autopsy study of 965 normal hearts. Mayo Clin Proc 1984; 59: 17-20.

[2]   Hausmann D, Mugge A, Becht I *et al.* Diagnosis of patent foramen ovale by transoesophageal echocardiography and association with cerebral and peripheral embolic events. Am J Cardiol 1992; 70: 668-672.

[3]   Anzola GP, Magoni M, Guindani M *et al.* Potential source of cerebral embolism in migraine with aura: a transcranial Doppler study. Neurology 1999; 52: 1622-1625.

[4]   Konstantinides S, Geibel A, Kasper W *et al.* Patent foramen ovale is an important predictor of adverse outcome in patients with major pulmonary embolism. Circulation 1998; 97: 1946-1951.

[5]   Mas J-L, Arquizan C, Lamy C *et al.* Recurrent cerebrovascular events associated with patent ovale, atrial septal aneurysm, or both. *NEJM* 2001; 345: 1740-1746.

[6]   Sacco RL, Ellenberg JH, Mohr JP, *et al.* Infarcts of undetermined cause: the NINCDS Stroke Data Bank. Ann Neurol 1989; 25: 382-390.

[7]   Wilmshurst PT, Pearson MJ, Walsh KP *et al.* Relationship between right-to-left shunts and cutaneous decompression illness. Clin Sci (Lond) 2001; 100(5): 539-42.

[8]   Giardini A, Donti A, Formigari A *et al.* Transcatheter patent foramen ovale closure mitigates aura migraine headaches abolishing spontaneous right-to-left shunting Am Heart J 2006; 151(4): 922.

[9]   Wilmshurst PT, Nightingale S. The role of cardiac and pulmonary pathology in migraine: a hypothesis. Headache. 2006; 46: 429-434.

[10]   Hildick-smith D, Behan M, Howarth P *et al.* Patent foramen ovale closure without echocardiographic control: use of "standby" intracardiac ultrasound. JACC Cardiovasc Interv 2008; 1(4): 387-91.

[11]   Homma S, Sacco RL, Di Tullio MR *et al.* Effect of medical treatment in stroke patients with patent foramen ovale. Patent foramen ovale and cryptogenic stroke study. Circulation 2002; 105: 2625-2631.

[12]   Devuyst G, Bogousslavsky J, Ruchat P *et al.* Prognosis after stroke followed by surgical closure of patent foramen ovale: a prospective follow-up study with brain MRI and simultaneous transesophageal and transcranial Doppler ultrasound. Neurology 1996; 47: 1162-1166.

[13]   Windecker S, Wahl A, Nedeltchev K *et al.* Comparison of medical treatment with percutaneous closure of patent foramen ovale in patients with cryptogenic stroke. J Am Coll Cardiol 2004; 44: 750-758.

[14]   Bridges ND, Hellenbrand W, Latson L *et al.* Transcatheter closure of patent foramen ovale after presumed paradoxical embolism. Circulation 1992; 86: 1902-1908.

[15]   Windecker S, Wahl A, Chatterjee T *et al.* Percutaneous closure of patent foramen ovale in patients with paradoxical embolism: long term risks of recurrent thrombotic events. Circulation 2000; 101: 893-898.

[16]   Morandi E, Anzola GP, Angeli S *et al.* Transcatheter closure of patent foramen ovale: a new migraine treatment? J Interv Cardiol. 2003; 16: 39-42.

[17]   Wilmshurst PT, Nightingale S, Walsh KP *et al.* Effect on migraine of closure of cardiac right-to-left shunts to prevent recurrence of decompression illness or stroke or for haemodynamic reasons. Lancet. 2000; 356: 1648-1651.

[18]   Dowson A, Mullen MJ, Peatfield R *et al.* A prospective, multicentre, double-blind, sham-controlled trial to evaluate the effectiveness of patent foramen ovale closure with STARFlex septal repair implant to resolve refractory migraine headache. Circulation. 2008; 117: 1397-1404.

[19]   Lock JE, Cockerham JT, Keane JF *et al.* Transcatheter umbrella closure of congenital heart defects. Circulation 1987; 75: 593-599.

CHAPTER 2

Percutaneous Closure of Atrial Septal Defects in Adults

David Hildick Smith[*]

Brighton & Sussex University Hospitals NHS Trust, Brighton, UK

Abstract: Percutaenous closure of atrial septal defects has become common place over the last 10 years. Patients with ASDs are at risk of atrial fibrillation and heart failure as the years progress and although little categorical evidence exists, expert consensus recommends closure of ASDs which are large enough to cause either symptoms or any change in right ventricular chamber size. The HELEX and in particular AMPLAZTER devices are well suited to device closure of ASDs, with high efficacy, low procedureal complication rates and very low long term complications rates. Patients with ASDS are now routinely considered for percutaneous rather than surgical closure of ASDs, though some requirement for surgery still exists amond patients with either very large ASDs or devicient inferior rims.

INTRODUCTION

Since percutaneous ASD closure was first conceived, the available devices, equipment and imaging techniques have improved to such an extent that the procedure can now be seen unequivocally as the treatment of choice in all but the largest atrial septal defects. Nonetheless, as with any new technology, pitfalls and problems remain. This chapter deals with the rationale, indications, procedural aspects and complications of percutaneous atrial septal defect closure.

RATIONALE

The natural history of ASD closure has been well documented, particularly during the 1960s and 1970s when surgical closure was the only alternative to medical therapy. It became clear that patients with significant ASDs tended to develop atrial fibrillation in their 40s, progressing to right heart failure and death in their 60s. Today it can be difficult to imagine this inevitable progression but many patients until 40 years ago followed exactly this path, and given that ASD has a prevalence of ~1% in the population, this was a significant cause of cardiovascular morbidity and mortality [1].

Left-to-right intracardiac flow through a significant atrial septal defect gradually overloads the right ventricle, which becomes enlarged. This facilitates tricuspid regurgitation through annular dilatation, further increasing the load on the expanding right atrium and leading, if uncorrected, to right heart failure.

INDICATIONS

The relative safety and simplicity of percutaneous ASD closure has gradually eroded the threshold at which ASD closure is considered appropriate. Historically, the traditional threshold for ASD closure was when the pulmonary to systemic shunt ratio was 2:1. This has now lessened to around 1.5:1, and indeed often the exact Qp:Qs is not measured [2].

In adult patients, the diagnosis of an atrial septal defect may be made due to investigation of lesion-specific symptoms, but equally, because of the high quality imaging techniques now available, the diagnosis is frequently "incidental". Patients who have an atrial septal defect of ≥1cm diameter are certainly at risk of atrial fibrillation and right heart volume overload in the fullness of time and should have the defect closed. Equally, patients who have a defect of 3mm are not at risk of haemodynamic complications, so the only indication to close would be due to paradoxical embolism. Individual operators will have different thresholds but in general it is reasonable to consider percutaneous closure for ASDs of >6 to 8mm.

Address correspondence to David Hildick Smith: Brighton & Sussex University Hospitals NHS Trust, Brighton, UK; E-mail: Smith@bsuh.nhs.uk

ANATOMICAL CONSIDERATIONS

There are many types of atrial septal defect and only the secundum ASD is suitable for percutaneous closure. Fortunately for the interventionist, the others, such as the sinus venosus, coronary sinus and ostium primum defects are not often encountered in adults. Anatomically, the key considerations are the size of the defect, the pulmonary venous drainage, proximity of the AV valves, the anterior superior aortic rim and the posterior inferior rim. Of these, it is the anterior superior rim which causes the greatest concern, as it is often deficient (<5mm) and frequently appears absent altogether in some planes. Given the fears of erosion, a balance has to be struck between oversizing the device and risking erosion, versus undersizing the device and risking either embolisation, or the need to upsize the device at the time of implantation (an expensive error). As a general rule, there is a school of thought which suggests that unless you have to upsize at implantation in 10% of cases, you are probably routinely oversizing your ASD closures. This is a good rule of thumb.

Although the deficient aortic rim is much discussed, deficiency of the posteroinferior IVC rim is of greater concern [3]. Firstly this is more difficult to diagnose, being less well visualised on transoesophageal echo unless particular efforts are made, and is therefore sometimes overlooked, and secondly in the absence of the inferior rim (in contrast to absence of the aortic rim) there is no associated structure to hold the device in place, and therefore the risk of embolisation is high. Intracardiac echo may delineate the inferior rim better than TOE in some cases.

IMAGING THE DEFECT

There are increasing numbers of procedures in interventional Cardiology where the interplay between the imaging physician and the implanting physician are critical, and percutaneous atrial septal defect closure is one of these. The diagnosis is usually first made, or hinted at, by transthoracic echocardiography. A more detailed scan, using transoesophageal echocardiography, ideally now with 3-D reconstruction, is then required to visualise the size, obliquity, rims and drainage related to the defect. Only one these are fully characterised can the closure procedure be planned appropriately.

Per-procedure imaging for percutaneous ASD closure is also vitally important. While simple patent foramen ovale defects can be successfully and uneventfully closed using contrast-guided angiography alone, the same is not true for atrial septal defects and per-procedure imaging is necessary to avoid incomplete coverage or risk of embolisation.

Operators have a choice of either intracardiac ultrasound (ICE) or transoesophageal echocardiography. The advantage of the former is that general anaesthesia is avoided, and therefore organisational difficulties are minimised. The advantage of the latter however is that the operator is freed to concentrate solely on aspects of implantation, without having to let go of the implantation equipment to optimise the ICE image. This can be particularly important during difficult implantations where either the angle of implant or the size of the defect are challenging.

THE PROCEDURE

The procedure is therefore usually done under general anaesthesia with transoesophageal echocardiographic guidance. Some operators have also done ASD closure under echo guidance alone, or fluoroscopy alone, but this is not advocated.

The right femoral vein is access with a large sheath (e.g. 11F). Pulmonary artery pressure may be recorded, and occasionally in older patients, arterial access is also gained, either to assess the coronary vasculature, or to allow monitoring of the left ventricular end-diastolic pressure during balloon occlusion of larger defects.

Crossing the defect is usually very straightforward using a guidewire through a multipurpose catheter. This exchange wire should then be positioned in the left or right upper pulmonary vein, taking care to avoid entering the left atrial appendage, which is a tracebulated structure with interwoven very thin areas.

Once the defect has been crossed, and this has been confirmed by echocardiography, a sizing balloon is usually used to assess the size and compliance of the defect. Some operators choose to size the defect simply from echocardiography, but this does not allow assessment of the rigidity of the margins.

Balloon measurement of the defect is usually now made to the "stop-flow" point. This means that colour flow is monitored as the balloon in inflated, and, rather than observe fluoroscopically for indentation of the balloon, the operator is advised by the echocardiographer when colour flow around the margins of the balloon has ceased. This is the stop-flow point, at which measurement of the diameter of the defect can be made both on echocardiography and fluoroscopy. 3-D imaging is helpful here, particularly with eccentric defects [4].

There is often disagreement between the fluoroscopic and echocardiographic measurements. It is therefore valuable to repeat these and come to a consensus agreement between the operators as to the correct size of the defect.

Once the size of the defect has been decided, the device must be chosen. Amplatzer devices are the only ones suitable for defects of 15mm or more. Below that, non-waisted devices such as the HELEX or BioSTAR can also be used. The size of the Amplatzer refers to the waist diameter. Beyond this there is a lip on the device for between 4 to 8mm either side, depending on the precise device. A 40mm device will therefore have a complete left atrial coverage of 56mm.

Selecting the exact device has become a thorny issue because of the rare cases of device erosion causing tamponade, sometimes fatal. The advice from the company expert consensus is not to oversize the device by more than 2mm, [5] however there is a body of opinion which suggests that splaying the device on the aortic rim is safer than having the device edges pointing directly onto it. Superior defects, where the roof of the left or right atrium may be eroded, are those in which care should be taken not to oversize the defect.

Implantation of the device may not be straightforward. The cable which holds the device in the catheter and prevents premature release is rigid and straightens the delivery sheath itself which is curved at its distal end. Depending on the angle of the inferior vena cava and the orientation of the interatrial septum, even simple-looking defects can sometimes be difficult to close.

Multiple techniques exist to facilitate the deployment of the device. The initial technique is to rotate the guide catheter clockwise toward the right upper pulmonary vein to try to align the left atrial disc with the interatrial septum. If this does not work, occasionally it is possible to rotate the guide catheter counterclockwise to wedge the left atrial disc against the most posterior aspect of the aorta as the rest of the device is then aligned with the defect and released. Opening the mid portion of the device such that the waist begins to sit in the defect itself is also often a successful ploy.

More advanced techniques for difficult lesions involved opening the left atrial disc in either the left or right upper pulmonary vein, then opening the right atrial disc at the level of the defect and then maintaining tension on the cable to release the left atrial disc from the pulmonary vein to snap into position at the interatrial septum. Alternatively, balloons can be used to keep the disc from prolapsing through the defect while the right atrial disc is released.

Once the device has been deployed, the echocardiographer needs to check in multiple planes that the device is firmly held and that there all important structures are free of the device, including the pulmonary veins, coronary sinus and anterior mitral valve leaflet. The inferior margin of the ASD should be clearly seen prior to release of the device.

For elderly patients, whose left ventricular compliance is reduced, left ventricular end-diastolic pressure should be monitored for at least ten minutes prior to release of the device. In some cases, end-diastolic pressure will rise to above 25mmHg. This is enough to induce pulmonary oedema. Under these circumstances, either the procedure can be terminated and the device withdrawn, or pharmacological measures can be taken to try to prevent pulmonary oedema while the heart adapts to the immediate change [6]. Equally, there has been concern regarding closure of defects in which pulmonary artery pressures are elevated. This fear however is misplaced. Patients who have pulmonary arterial systolic pressures of <75% systemic can have their atrial septal defect closed without concern, and with good clinical results [7].

COMPLICATIONS

Procedural complications are relatively rare. Arteriovenous malformation occurs due to inadvertent arterial and venous puncture at the groin when the artery and vein lie superimposed. Device embolisation at the time of the procedure is relatively rare, with an incidence of 1-2% [8]. When this occurs, the device usually embolises to the pulmonary artery, but occasionally to the left ventricle. From the pulmonary artery, the device can be snared using a goose-neck snare, and can usually be retrieved into the guide catheter in the right atrium. From the systemic circulation, retrieval is more difficult. The device may become lodged in the mitral valve apparatus, in which case it may be retrieved transseptally, or may come to lie in the ascending aorta, in which case large bore arterial access is required to grasp the device and resheath it.

Erosion is much feared but does not usually occur early. Patients may represent months after the initial procedure, either with acute tamponade, or with cardiac death. Similarly, embolisation can occur late, though it is more usual for this to occur within 24 hours of the implantation procedure.

Atrial rhythm disturbances are common in the early post-procedure phase. Sustained atrial fibrillation may occur in up to 5% of cases. By 6 months post-procedure however, ongoing atrial rhythm disturbance is rare [9].

Migraine occurs sporadically in up to 2% of patients during the first six months post-implantation. This is thought to relate to platelet activation on the left atrial disc, but no clear pathophysiological mechanism has been established.

CONCLUSIONS

The vast majority of atrial septal defects can now be closed non-surgically. Percutaneous atrial septal defect closure is an effective and safe procedure when undertaken by suitably trained physicians. Procedural risks are low and long-term outcomes are good.

REFERENCES

[1]   Campbell M. Natural history of atrial septal defect. Br Heart J 1970; 32(6): 820-6.

[2]   Gatzoulis MA, Redington AN, Somerville J, Shore DF. Should atrial septal defects in adults be closed? Ann Thorac Surg 1996; 61(2): 657-9.

[3]   Mathewson JW, Bichell D, Rothman A, Ing FF. Absent posteroinferior and anterosuperior atrial septal defect rims: Factors affecting nonsurgical closure of large secundum defects using the Amplatzer occluder. J Am Soc Echocardiogr 2004; 17(1): 62-9.

[4]   Lodato JA, Cao QL, Weinert L, Sugeng L, Lopez J, Lang RM, *et al.* Feasibility of real-time three-dimensional transoesophageal echocardiography for guidance of percutaneous atrial septal defect closure. Eur J Echocardiogr 2009; 10(4): 543-8.

[5]   Amin Z, Hijazi ZM, Bass JL, Cheatham JP, Hellenbrand WE, Kleinman CS. Erosion of Amplatzer septal occluder device after closure of secundum atrial septal defects: review of registry of complications and recommendations to minimize future risk. Catheter Cardiovasc Interv 2004; 63(4): 496-502.

[6]   Schubert S, Peters B, Abdul-Khaliq H, Nagdyman N, Lange PE, Ewert P. Left ventricular conditioning in the elderly patient to prevent congestive heart failure after transcatheter closure of atrial septal defect. Catheter Cardiovasc Interv 2005; 64(3): 333-7.

[7]   Balint OH, Samman A, Haberer K, Tobe L, McLaughlin P, Siu SC, *et al.* Outcomes in patients with pulmonary hypertension undergoing percutaneous atrial septal defect closure. Heart 2008; 94(9): 1189-93.

[8]   Tomar M, Radhakrishnan S, Shrivastava S. Transcatheter closure of fossa ovalis atrial septal defect: a single institutional experience. Indian Heart J 2006; 58(4): 325-9.

[9]   Giardini A, Donti A, Sciarra F, Bronzetti G, Mariucci E, Picchio FM. Long-term incidence of atrial fibrillation and flutter after transcatheter atrial septal defect closure in adults. Int J Cardiol 2009; 134(1): 47-51.

CHAPTER 3

Transcatheter Aortic Valve Implantation

Isma Rafiq[1,*] and Cameron G. Densem[2,*]

[1]Papworth Hospital, Cambridge, UK and [2]Papworth Hospital, Cambridge, UK

Abstract: Transcatheter aortic valve implantation is an emerging technology which has brought promise for high risk patients with symptomatic severe aortic stenosis deemed unsuitable for surgery. Aortic stenosis is a common valvular problem representing 4.6% of population aged > 75 [1]. This presents a long term public problem as the prevalence of the disease increase with age so does other morbidities which deem some portion of this group inoperable due to increased surgical morbidity and mortality. First transcatheter aortic valve was implanted by Cribier in 2002 [2]. The initial results were promising but antegrade technique was challenging which led to innovation of a flexible retrograde delivery system with improved procedural outcome [3]. To avoid access problems and provide more stability, transapical approach was developed. They are two systems available, the Edwards SAPIEN valve is a bovine pericardium prosthesis mounted on a balloon-expandable stent that is placed in the subcoronary position and the CoreValve Revalving system compromises of self expanding bioprosthetic valve with a ninitol frame{2}[4]. The initial and median results have been promising whilst the long term results are awaited. With development of new delivery system and devices, the technology will promise a better procedural and clinical effective outcome.

INTRODUCTION

Transcatheter aortic valve implantation (TAVI) is an exciting novel technique for patients with aortic valve disease at higher than average risk from open surgical intervention. Plain balloon aortic valvuloplasty was the first transcatheter technique for aortic valve stenosis. This procedure is, however, palliative as the stenosis always recurs between 6 and 24 months. A percutaneous approach to aortic valve implantation was first explored by Andersen as a translation of stent technology [5, 6]. Later Cribier designed and implanted the first transcatheter aortic valve prosthesis into a human in 2002 after animal trials [7, 3]. Using a balloon expandable system *via* a transvenous antegrade approach the initial results were promising but the procedures were challenging and time consuming with a significant risk of complications, especially to the mitral valve [8]. The next innovation was a transarterial retrograde approach pioneered by Webb [3]. This improved procedural outcome and has allowed the technique to rapidly spread worldwide since the first successful case in 2004. A significant proportion of patients were not suitable for a transfemoral approach due to issues with the peripheral vasculature. The transapical method, prosthetic insertion directly through the left ventricular apex *via* a limited thoracotomy overcomes any problems related to the aorto-iliac vessels. A second aortic valve implant, the self expanding ninitol CoreValve, was introduced to clinical practice in 2005 [4]. This can be also be implanted *via* a retrograde transarterial approach and provides a viable alternative. Numerous other devices are currently in development and will enter the clinical arena within the next few years.

TAVI procedures have necessitated a new way of working. Close collaboration between cardiologists and surgeons as part of a multidisciplinary team is essential. All techniques and prostheses continue to be modified. This will improve the peri-procedural success rate as well as safety, opening up the possibility of treatment to a wider population. Longer term and randomised trial data against a surgical approach are awaited.

BACKGROUND – AORTIC VALVE STENOSIS AND AORTIC VALVE REPLACEMENT

Valvular heart disease is an increasing public health problem as the population ages around the world. Aortic valve stenosis is the most common form in adults; [1]. in populations over 75 years of age the prevalence may be as high as 4.6%. The vast majority are degenerative in aetiology (Fig. **1a** and **1b**). Untreated cases are associated with an incidence of sudden death of 10-15% per year with an average survival of 2-3 years [9].

Intervention for aortic valve stenosis is generally indicated with the onset of symptoms, angina, breathlessness, syncope, exertional dizziness, and/or the development of left ventricular dysfunction particularly if asymptomatic. Trans-sternal aortic valve replacement surgery with cardiopulmonary bypass is considered to be the gold standard

*Address correspondence to Isma Rafiq and Cameron G Densem: Papworth Hospital, Cambridge, UK; E-mails: ismach@doctors.org; Cameron.Densem@papworth.nhs.uk

therapy (Fig. **2a** and **b**). However several factors increase the risk of operative mortality; reduced left ventricular function, age, the presence of coronary disease and co-morbidities such as significant renal dysfunction, and debilitating cerebrovascular disease. To reduce the insult and morbidity of trans-sternal surgery minimal access aortic valve replacement has been developed but his still requires cardiopulmonary bypass and a static heart.

The Euroheart survey has famously shown that one third of patients, despite having severe symptomatic aortic valve stenosis, do not undergo surgery. In North America this rate may be higher. This is due to a combination of reasons. Some patients are deemed to be of too high operative risk by their physician, cardiologist or cardiothoracic surgeon. Some may simply live within their symptoms whilst others do not wish to undergo major heart surgery late in life.

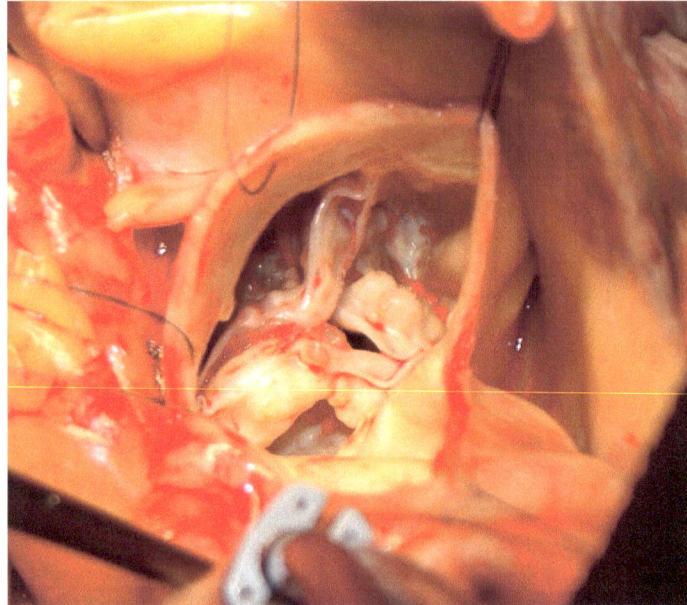

Figure 1a: Degenerated Stenotic Aortic Valve Prior to Surgical Excision.

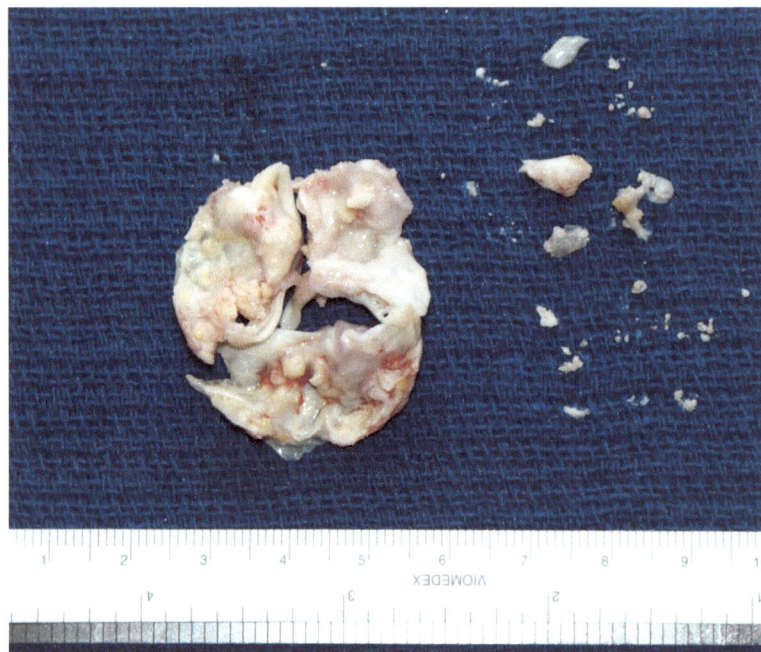

Figure 1b: The Valve of Fig. **1a** After Excision.

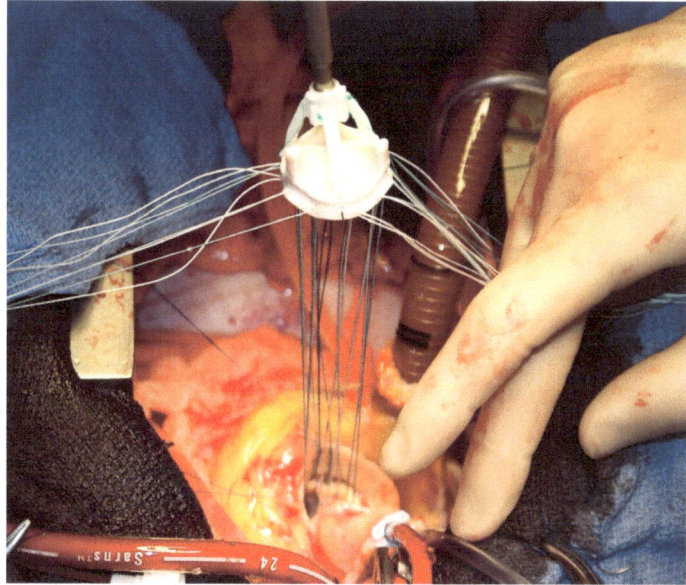

Figure 2a: Biological Aortic Valve Prosthesis Being Lowered in to Position.

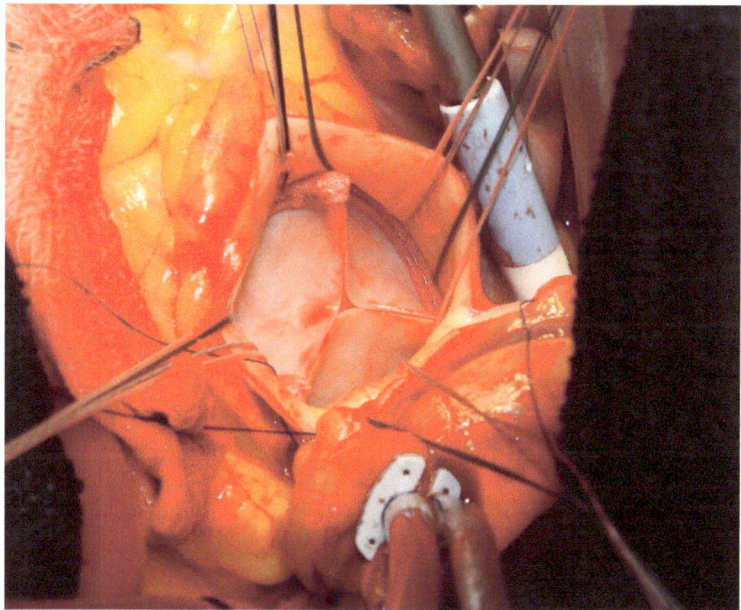

Figure 2b: A Biological Aortic Valve Prosthesis In-Situ.

CLINICAL INDICATIONS FOR TAVI

TAVI was developed as an alternative to surgery but also as a way of improving the longer term outcome after balloon aortic valvuloplasty. The latter is a palliative procedure reserved for those not suitable for the gold standard therapy of surgical aortic valve replacement. TAVI, therefore, began as a palliative procedure on a compassionate basis. With development its application has now extended to include patients at high risk from conventional surgery, and not just those who have been turned down [10]. More recently the National Institute of Clinical Excellence (NICE) has restricted the use of TAVI to selected patients [11].

Patient selection should be ideally carried out by a multidisciplinary team including interventional cardiologists, cardiac surgeons, and cardiac anaesthetists and imaging specialists e.g. Echocardiologist, CT and MRI radiologists [10]. Commonly adopted clinical criteria for eligibility are summarised in Table **1**.

Table 1: Clinical indicators for TAVI

Suitability Criteria
1. Logistic Euroscore > 20 or STS risk calculator score > 10
2. Refused Surgery by Two Surgeons
3. Previous sternotomy and patent coronary artery bypass graft
4. Severe Respiratory disease
5. Radiation treatment of the sternum
Potential indications for TAVI
1. Logistic Euroscore >20 or STS risk calculator score >10
2. Refused surgery by two independent cardiothoracic surgeons
3. Previous sternotomy and patent coronary artery bypass grafts, especially the internal mammary vessels
4. Severe co-morbid disease e.g. renal failure, severe lung disease
5. Prior radiotherapy of the mediastinum.
6. Porcelain aorta

Patients with previous sternotomies and patent bypass grafts lend themselves very well to these techniques. Redo sternotomy carries increased risk or mortality and morbidity especially if the internal internal mammary graft remains patent.

CONTRAINDICATIONS FOR TAVI

There are a number of relative and absolute contraindications to TAVI which are summarised in Table **2**. Technical and clinical considerations aside thought should also be given to the functional capacity of the patient. Patients who have been poorly functional and unable to conduct activities of daily living for some time are unlikely to make significant gains in quality of life afterwards. Likewise patients who are severely symptomatic from co-morbidities, for example severe debilitating lung disease are unlikely to benefit overall from relief of left ventricular outflow tract obstruction depending on their presenting symptom.

Table 2: Some of the common contraindications to TAVI

1.	Unsuitable sizing of aortic annulus or root, specific for an individual device.
2.	Non Valvular, congenital or non-calcific aortic stenosis.
3.	Intra-cardiac mass, thrombus, vegetation
4.	Active infection or endocarditis
5.	High ischaemic burden
6.	Myocardial infarction within the last month
7.	Double or Triple Valve Disease
8.	Very severe ventricular dysfunction
9.	Left ventricular apical thrombus, especially if a transapical approach
10.	Recent pulmonary emboli or cerebrovascular accident
11.	Co-morbid disease which would independently limit prognosis

METHODS OF TRANSCATHETER AORTIC VALVE IMPLANTATION

TAVI has a number of potential advantages over a formal surgical approach. These are summarised in Table **3**.

Table 3: Potential Advantages of Transcatheter Aortic Valve Implantation over Conventional Surgery

1. Lower risk for selected patients
2. Faster Recovery
3. Avoidance of cardiopulmonary bypass
4. Avoidance of aortic cross clamping
5. Shorter ITU and overall hospital stay
6. Shorter intubation times
7. Earlier mobilisation
8. Avoidance of sternal complications
9. Avoidance of injury to patent bypass grafts

Two different types of prosthesis are currently commercially available; the Sapien valve (Edwards Lifesciences Inc., IR, USA) and the CoreValve Revalving system (Medtronic, MN, USA). In the next few years an increased range of devices are likely to become available.

THE EDWARDS SAPIEN VALVE

The current Sapien valve is a balloon expandable unidirectional trileaflet tissue valve with polyethylene terephthalate cuff modified from the original Cribier prosthesis. It is comprised of 3 leaflets fashioned from bovine pericardium suspended within a stainless steel stent (Fig. **3**). It is designed to be positioned and subsequently deployed within the aortic valve annulus in the subcoronary position either by a retrograde or an antegrade approach. It is soon to be available in a variety of diameters but early operators had the choice of 23 or 26mm devices [11, 12]. These valves can be deployed within an annulus ranging from 18mm to 25mm in diameter [11].

The device comes with an introducer kit which includes a crimping tool to symmetrically compress the prosthesis on to the balloon, a steerable delivery catheter, a set of hydrophilic dilators for a transfemoral approach and a wide bore introducer sheath. The valve is preserved in low concentration solutions of buffered glutaraldehyde which must be washed off prior to implantation (Fig. **4**).

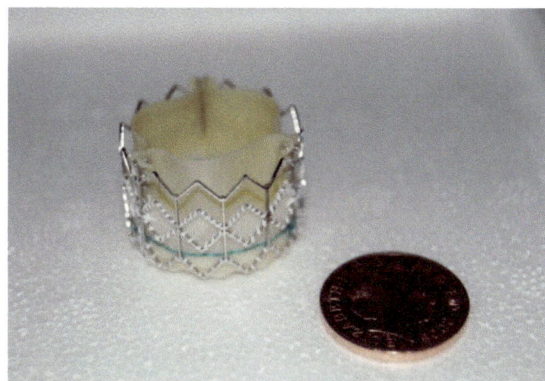

Figure 3: Sapien Balloon Expandable Transcatheter Aortic Valve. A British One penny piece has been included for scale (similar in size to an American one cent coin).

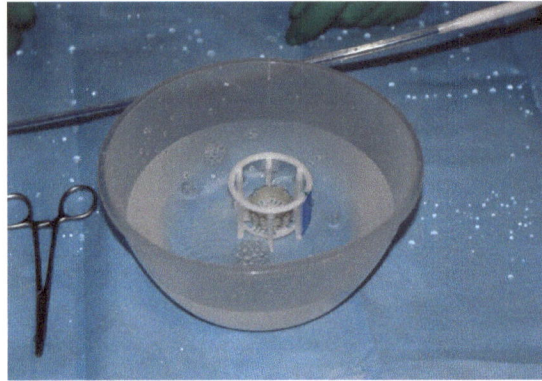

Figure 4: Initial Preparation of the Valve Involves Washing.

THE COREVALVE REVALVING SYSTEM

The bioprosthetic CoreValve device consists of a trileaflet porcine pericardial tissue valve mounted and sutured within a self-expanding 50mm nitinol stent frame [4]. A Corevalve has three distinct portions. The lower segment exerts a high radial force that pushes the calcified leaflets aside. The central portion carries the bioprosthetic valve and tapers to avoid the coronary ostia and the upper part flares to fixate and stabilise the deployed prosthetic valve in the ascending aorta to prevent migration and embolization.

The CoreValve design provides several advantages that facilitate device deployment and reliable implantation [13]. Firstly, a certain deployment error margin because of the larger size relative to the Edwards system. Secondly, self centring properties. Thirdly, beneficial anchoring characteristics in the native valve area as well as the ascending aorta and finally the capacity for device retrieval after partial implantation of the first two-thirds of the prosthesis. Having deployed the distal two-thirds of the prosthesis the valve is already sufficiently functioning, whereas the device position can still be adjusted or the device can be removed completely. The CoreValve, however, can only be positioned using retrograde techniques. Once in place within the stenosed native valve the overlying sheath is removed whilst maintaining position of the prosthesis. As the device is revealed it expands back to its engineered size and shape.

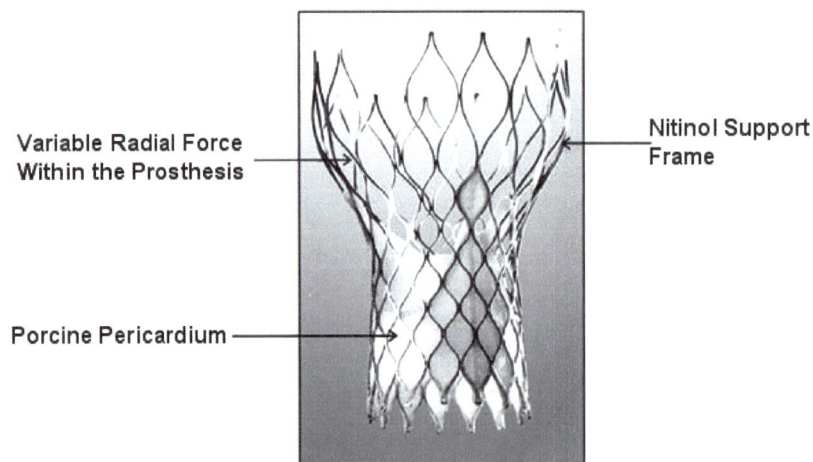

Figure 5: Corevalve Revalving Self Expandable System (courtesy of the Wythenshawe (Manchester) TAVI team.

METHODS OF TRANSCATHETER AORTIC VALVE IMPLANTATION

A more detailed description of implant methodology is described later in the chapter. Fig. **6** highlights the traditional routes of TAVI.

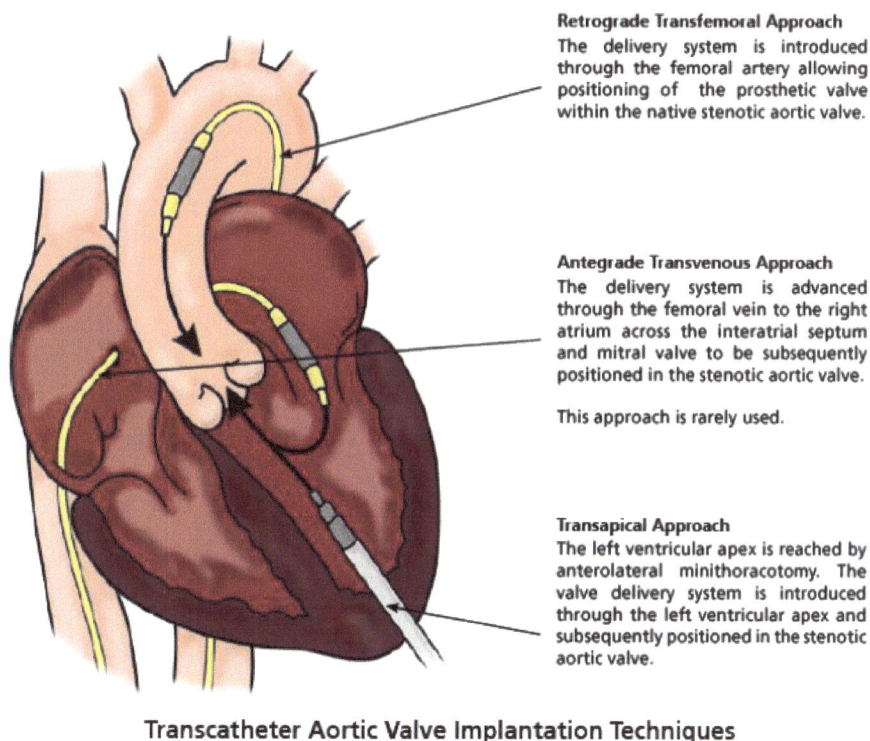

Transcatheter Aortic Valve Implantation Techniques

Figure 6: Traditional Methods of Transcatheter Aortic Valve Implantation.

1. The Antegrade Transvenous Approach

This was the first technique of TAVI within humans as described by Cribier [2, 8]. Access to the circulation was through the femoral vein. The left atrium was then accessed *via* the inferior vena cava, right atrium and a trans-septal puncture. A balloon tipped catheter was used to cross the mitral valve in to the left ventricle and subsequently through the aortic valve. This allowed delivery of a guide wire which was subsequently externalised *via* a femoral artery. This becomes the rail for delivery of the aortic prosthesis. The main advantage of this technique is that the femoral vein can accommodate large catheters and it is easy to secure haemostasis [2, 8, 14]. This technique is now, however, rarely used because of time consumption, technical difficulties and the potential for mitral valve injury by the wire [15].

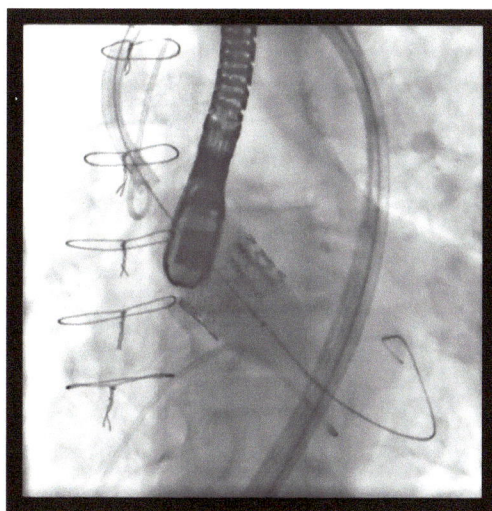

Figure 7: Deployment of a Transfemoral Balloon Expandable Transcatheter Prosthesis.

2. The Retrograde Approach

Usually this technique involves a trans-femoral approach but trans-iliac, trans-aortic or trans-subclavian methods can also be adopted. By whichever method the aortic prosthesis is delivered retrogradely across the stenosed valve. It can either be *via* an open surgical cut down technique or with experience as a purely percutaneous procedure. The latter depends on anatomy and operator choice. Either common femoral artery can be chosen depending on the vascular anatomy [3, 8].

Once access is achieved, a guide wire is advanced retrogradely into the aorta and manipulated across the aortic valve under fluoroscopy. The ilio-femoral artery is then dilated to accommodate the delivery sheath. Both commercially available valve systems can be used *via* this approach.

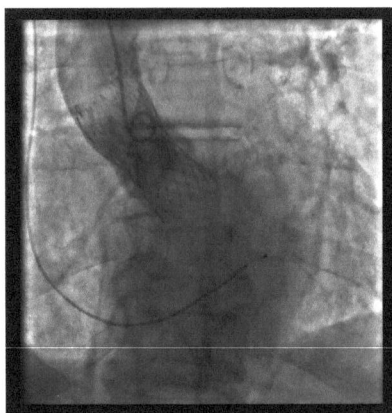

Figure 8: A Deploymed of a Transfemoral Corevalve Prosthesis (Courtesy of Dr David Hildick-Smith).

3. The Transapical Approach

TAVI equipment is large calibre and relatively stiff. As such the chosen peripheral vessels need to be adequately sized to accommodate. The transapical approach is the alternative technique when a retrograde method is not technically feasible [16, 17].

The cardiac apex is localised by using transthoracic echocardiogram, and a submammary mini-thoracotomy is performed, 5-7cm in length. The pericardium is opened to expose the apex of the heart. Pledgeted sutures are initially placed in the left ventricular apex or anterior wall. The apex is punctured with a seldinger needle and a guide wire is introduced into the left ventricle. The guide wire is directed anterogradely through the left ventricular outflow tract across the native aortic valve into the ascending and descending aorta. The needle is removed and a coronary catheter is passed over the wire. The initial wire is then exchanged for an amplatz extra stiff wire over which is then passed a sheath for BAV or the Ascendra system for TAVI. The apex is dilated until it is suitable for the passage of the delivery catheter. After completion of the procedure the sheath is removed and the pledgeted sutures are tied to close the left ventriculotomy. A left chest drain is left in the pleura and the thoracotomy is closed [18].

A comparison of the Transfemoral and Transapical approaches are presented in Table **4**.

Table 4: Comparison of the Advantages and Disadvantages of the Two Common Techniques

Transfemoral Technique	**Transapical Technique**
No Thoracotomy	Fewer vascular access problems
No distortion of apical anatomy	Delivery system size less important
Smaller delivery sheath	Shorter delivery system
General anaesthesia is optional	Conversion open surgery easier
Potential shorter ITU and hospital stay.	Avoidance of atherosclerotic arteries

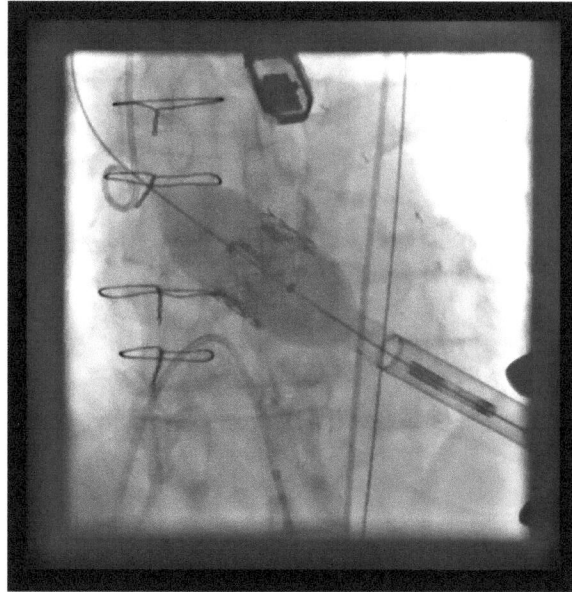

Figure 9: Deployment of a Transapical Balloon Expandable Valve.

PREOPERATIVE ASSESSMENT OF PATIENTS FOR TRANSCATHETER AORTIC VALVE IMPLANTATION

1. Patient Selection

Patients should be considered for TAVI by a multidisciplinary team adhering to the criteria listed in Table **1**. If a patient is clinically eligible they should then undergo a series of investigations to guide risk and the technical suitability for TAVI [19]. as described below.

2. Echocardiographic Assessment

A detailed description of the echocardiographic assessment of aortic valve physiology and anatomy is beyond the realms of this chapter. There are, however, specific indices which are of particular interest to the TAVI operator.

a. Severity of Aortic Valve Stenosis

Echocardiography is initially essential to confirm the presence of degenerative calcific severe aortic valve stenosis (Fig. **10**). Generally a peak gradient over 70mmHg, a mean gradient over 40mmHg (in the context of preserved left ventricular function) and/or a valve area of less than 1 cm^2 are accepted indicators of severe stenosis (Fig. **11**). A transoesophageal study may be required if non-diagnostic transthoracic pictures are acquired (Fig. **12**).

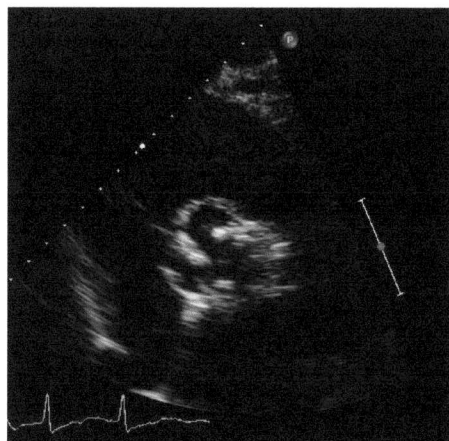

Figure 10: Transthoracic Short Axis View Showing a Heavily Calcified Trileaflet Aortic Valve.

As the field develops the indication is likely to extend to senile degenerative aortic valve regurgitation. With current technology it would be important to exclude an underlying dilative aortic pathology as this may lead to device embolization should it continue to progress.

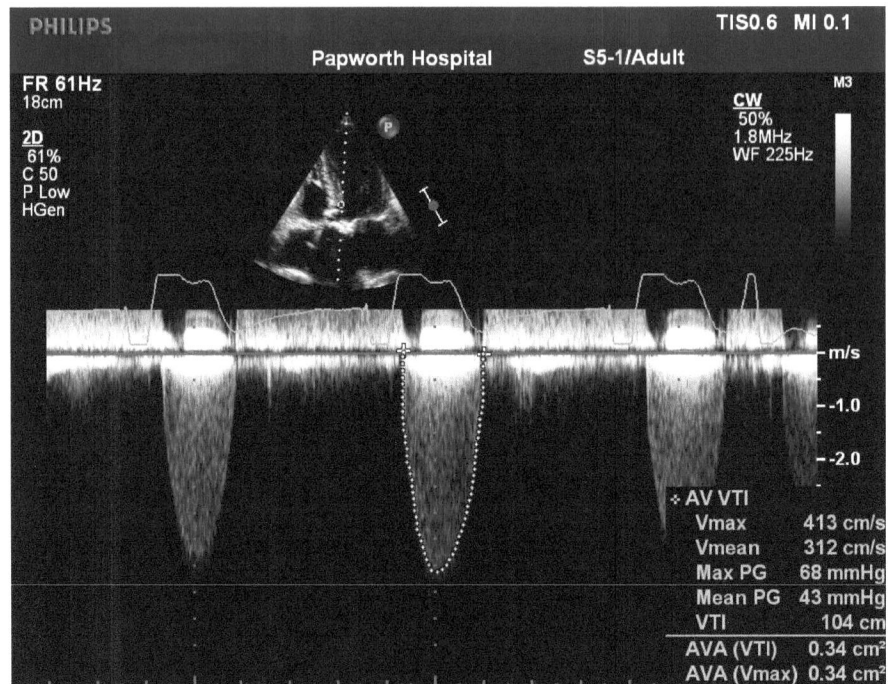

Figure 11: Continuous Wave Doppler Pressure Trace Across a Severely Stenosed Aortic Valve with a Valve Area of 0.34cm2.

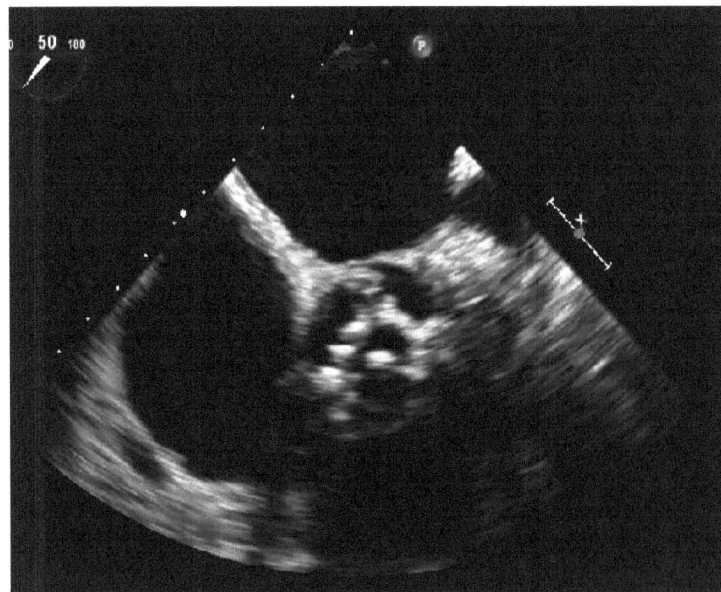

Figure 12: Transoesophageal View of a Trileaflet Aortic Valve Showing Stenotic Degeneration.

b. Measurement of Aortic Valve Annulus

Due to the current size limitations of the technology it is essential that the aortic valve annulus is carefully assessed to ensure it falls within the desired range for the chosen prosthesis. The Edwards system requires an 18 to 25mm diameter, and the CoreValve system 20 to 27mm. Any smaller and there is a risk of annular perforation and aortic rupture as well as device failure due to poor expansion and leaflet function. For larger annulae there is a risk of device embolization. It is the interaction of the outward radial force of the stent frame against the degenerated calcific nodular native aortic valve that holds these devices in place. If borderline measurements or suboptimal views are obtained with a transthoracic echocardiogram a transoesophageal study is recommended to obtain the definitive measurement (Fig. **13**).

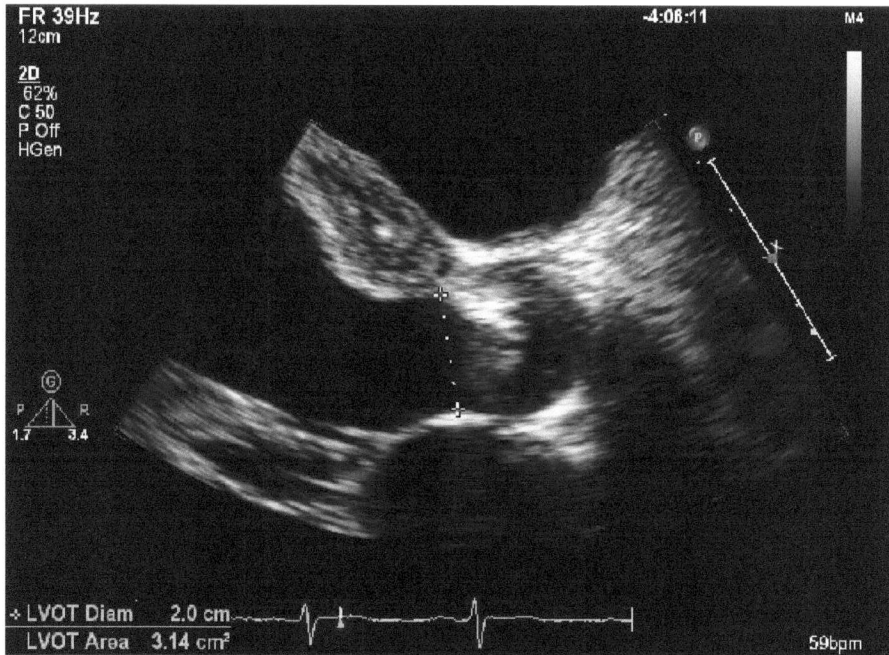

Figure 13: Transthoracic Measurement of the Aortic Annulus (2.0cm) taken from the Insertion Points of the Leaflets.

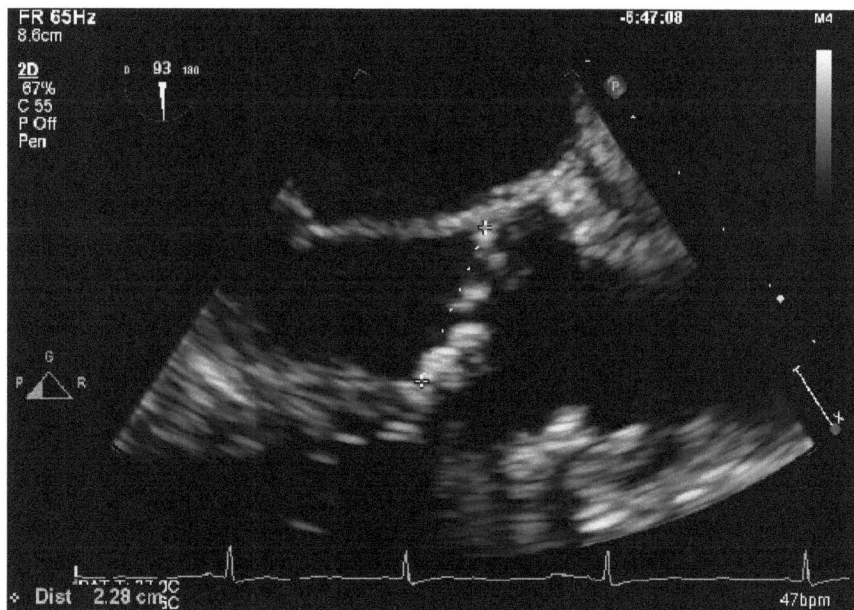

Figure 14: Using Transoesophageal Imaging for Accurate Annular Measuring.

c. Degree and Localisation of Leaflet Calcification

A valve which is only mildly calcified is more difficult to see by fluoroscopy thus making placement that little more difficult. Conversely severe nodular calcification will influence the degree of paraprosthetic leak after a successful implant.

d. Aortic Sinus and Root Measurements

These are critical for the CoreValve Revalving system as the interaction with the aortic root influences the centring, orientation and support of the prosthesis. The sinotubular junction can be no greater than 43mm in diameter for 29mm device and 40mm for the 26mm device. See Fig. **15** for an example of some of the measurements taken.

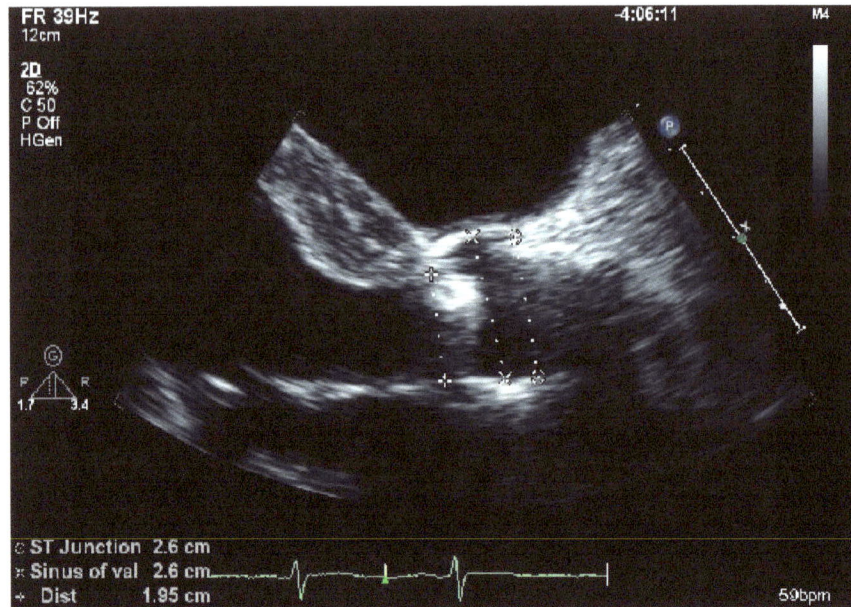

Figure 15: Measurement of the Aortic Valve and Sinsuses.

e. Assessment of Left Ventricular Outflow Tract and Position of the Coronary Ostia

A prominent septal bulge may interfere with accurate device placement leading to upward displacement (Fig. **16**). Likewise above the aortic valve coronary ostia which are visualised to be low within the aortic sinuses may be at risk of occlusion with valve implant. The latter is probably best assessed fluoroscopically or at the time of the preliminary BAV.

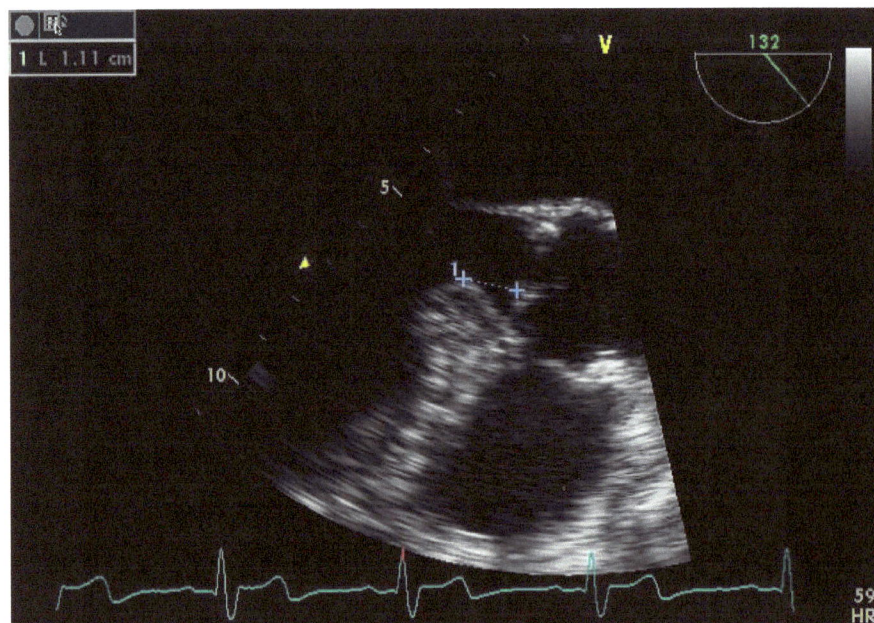

Figure 16: A Prominent Septal Bulge Just under the Aortic Annulus may Interfere with Deployment of the Device.

f. Left Ventricular Function and Systolic and Diastolic Dimensions

Poor left ventricular function is an adverse risk factor for aortic valve intervention. It may also push decision making towards a Transfemoral approach rather than disrupting the apex.

g. Assessment of Concomitant Valve Disease

The presence of severe concurrent valve disease may lean decision making towards an open procedure should it be not amenable to transcatheter repair. Severe untreated non aortic valve disease may hamper the clinical benefit expected from a TAVI.

h. Pulmonary Artery Pressure

A high pulmonary pressure contributes to the Euroscore and well be a risk factor for TAVI in the same way as for open surgery.

i. Exclusion of Left Ventricular Apical Thrombus

This is particularly important if a Transapical approach is planned for obvious reasons (Fig. **17**).

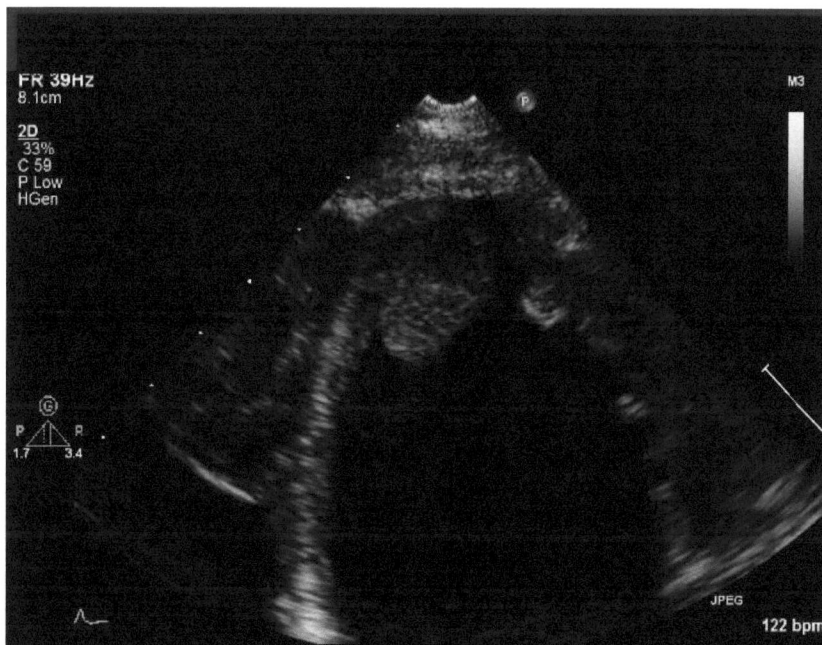

Figure 17: Evidence of Large Thrombus Within a Dilated Ventricle Which Would Contraindicate a Transapical Approach. (Courtesy of Dr R. Rusk).

3. Coronary Angiography and Aortography

Coronary angiography is essential to document the presence and extent of coronary artery disease. Should critical disease be seen percutaneous coronary angioplasty may be recommended prior to the TAVI. Large territories of poorly vascularised, yet viable, myocardium is a risk factor for an adverse outcome with TAVI. If disease is not amenable to angioplasty this may push the decision back towards open surgery.

Localisation of the left and right coronary ostia relative to the aortic valve leaflets is also essential. This is more important for the left main stem as generally the right coronary ostium sits higher within the aortic root. This distance is highly variable being independent of patient's stature. With device implantation if the left main stem is low lying, the native left aortic valve leaflet can occlude it leading to severe myocardial ischaemia. This is less of a concern in the presence of patent bypass grafts. It is important to define the distance between the inferior aspect of the sinus of valsalva and inferior aspect of the lowest coronary ostia before implanting the prosthetic valve.

Aortography defines the anatomical orientation of the aortic root, arch and descending aorta (Fig. **18**). A transverse aortic root has been a previous relative contraindication for a transfemoral approach but this is less of a problem with newer technology. Its is also useful to document the degree of baseline aortic regurgitation. In a patient with poor LV function and a large ischaemic burden they may struggle to tolerate an increased degree of regurgitation if a balloon valvuloplasty is performed with subsequent failure to place a prosthesis.

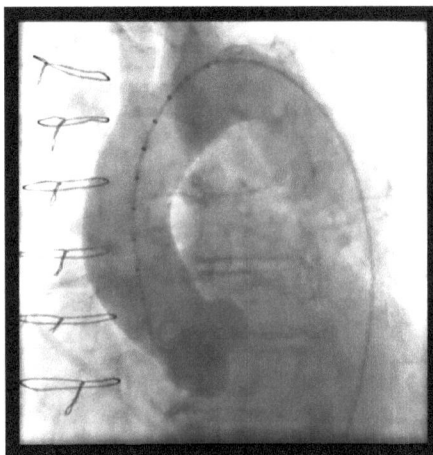

Figure 18: Aortogram with a Graded Pigtail (1cm Separation of Gold Markers) Showing the Relative Position of the Coronaries to the Plane of the Aortic Valve Annulus.

4. Peripheral Angiography

This is essential if a transiliofemoral approach is planned. All delivery equipment is bulky and large calibre. Angiography with quantitation is required to ensure adequate sizing of the peripheral vessels and to ensure an absence of significant tortuosity (Figs. **19** and **20**). A graded pigtail catheter is placed in the abdominal aorta just below the renal arteries. It is then important to document the arteries bilaterally all the way to the superficial femoral arteries. In some circumstances patients may be more suitable for a retroperitoneal transiliac approach rather than a transfemoral approach in order to avoid significant more distal vascular disease.

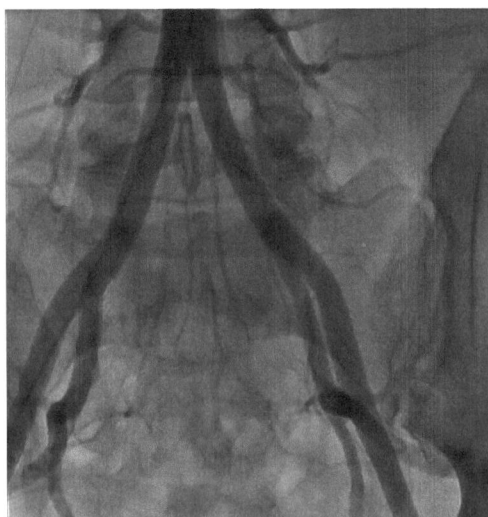

Figure 19: Very Favourable Straight Large Calibre Iliac Arteries for Transfemoral Approach.

5. Right Heart Catheterisation

This is useful in some patients with evidence of pulmonary hypertension with or without other valvular heart disease.

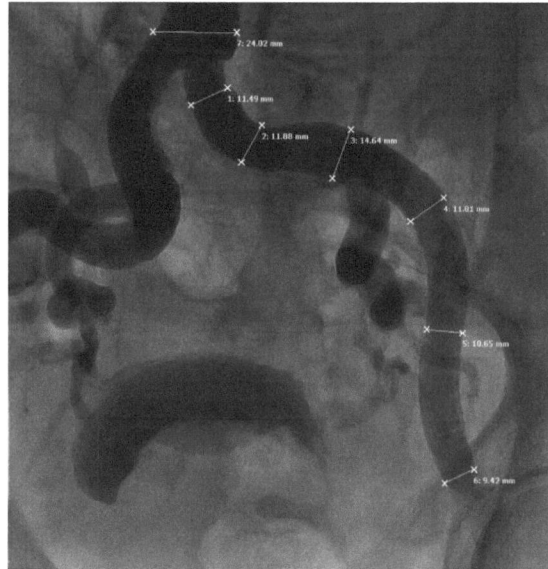

Figure 20: Peripheral Angiogram Showing Measurement of the Left Iliac Artery. The Graded pigtail Catheter with 1 cm Spaced Gold Markers can be Seen in the Right Iliac Artery. The Left Side is more Suitable for TAVI than the Right as it is Straighter.

6. Contrast CT Angiography

Computed tomographic angiography is essential for two main reasons. Firstly, if a transapical approach is planned it allows another method to exclude left ventricular thrombus. This is more likely to be present in the setting of reduced left ventricular function.

Secondly, for a transfemoral approach it is essential to assess again the calibre of the iliofemoral arteries looking specifically for the localisation and degree of calcification. The finding of severe abdominal aortic disease is also important particularly if anuerysmal or thrombotic.

The principle indication for TAVI may be a porcelain aorta. CT imaging allows interrogation of the extent and confluence of the aortic wall calcification.

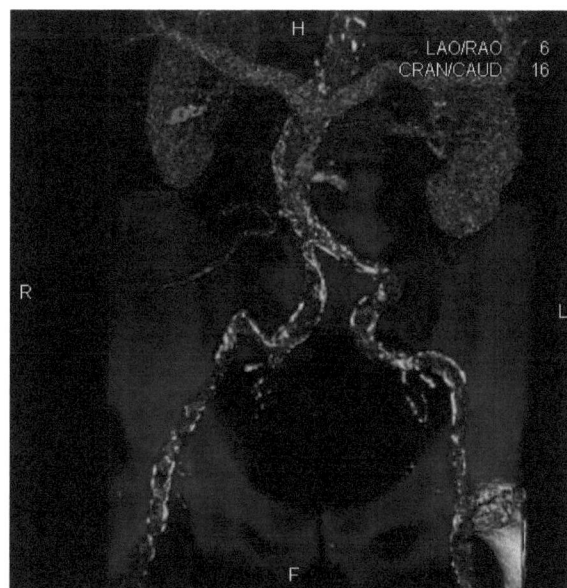

Figure 21: Peripheral CT Angiogram Showing Tortuous and Calcified Vessels. This Patient is a Less Likely Candidate for a Transfemoral Approach.

7. Electrocardiography

Conduction disease is more prevalent in patients with aortic valve disease. Should severe AV block be demonstrated on a screening ECG a pre-emptive permanent pacemaker may be advisable. The pattern of right bundle branch and left axis deviation may have an increased risk of perioperative complete heart block (Figs. **22** and **23**).

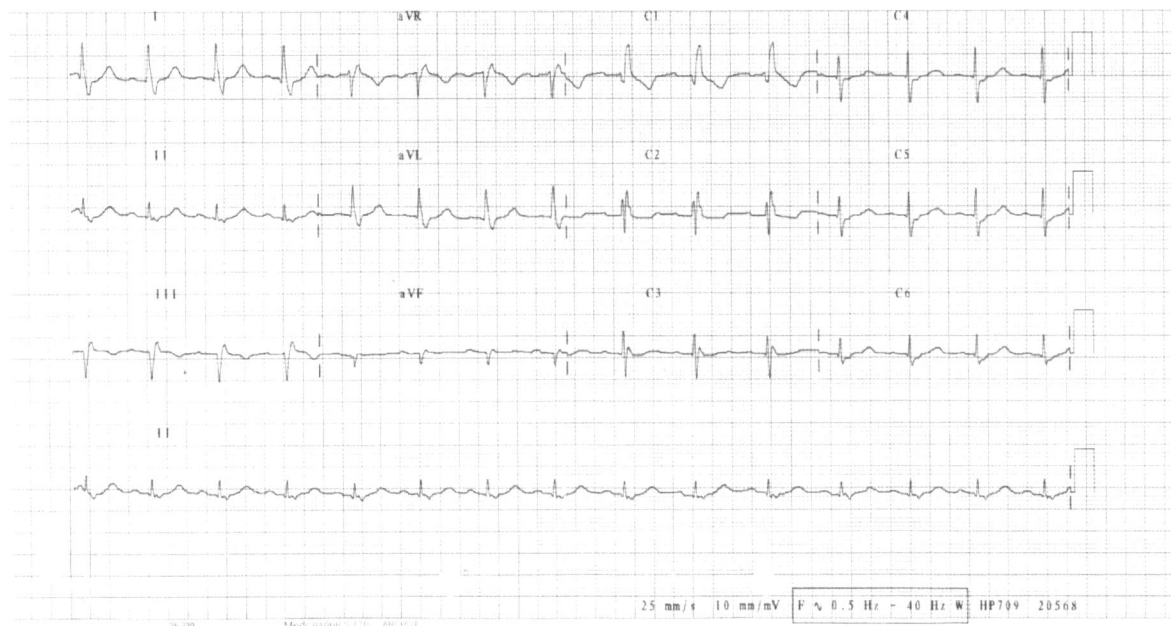

Figure 22: Baseline Electrocardiogram Showing a Trifascicular Block with Right Bundle and Left Anterior Hemiblock Dysfunction.

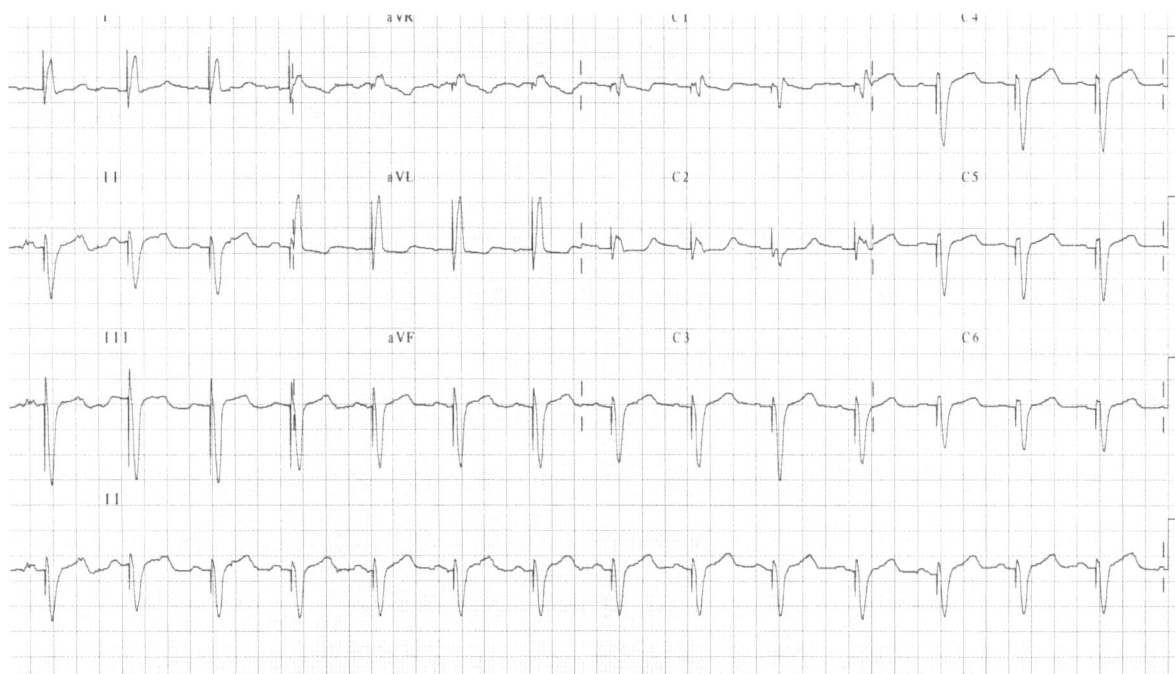

Figure 23: The Same Patient Demonstrating Trifascicular Block Post Operatively Demonstrating Permanent Pacing.

8. Magnetic Resonance Imaging

MRI has little role in TAVI assessment at the moment. As the indications for TAVI develop MRI will become useful in patients who have had previous mitral valve surgery, either a ring or prosthesis. There is concern that should the mitral and aortic prostheses rub together this may disrupt the intervening tissue. Technically, for a balloon mounted device as the balloon expands against a rigid mitral valve ring it may be forced to embolize cranially. An MRI would be able to visualise the plane of both the aortic and mitral valve annulae (Fig. **24a** and **b**). If they are offset by, for example greater than 7mm, a TAVI would be more likely to be successful.

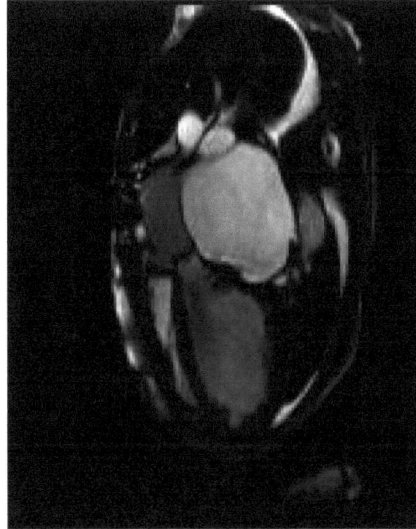

Figure 24a: Cardiac Magnetic Resonance Imaging to Show the Relative Planes of the Aortic and Prosthetic Valve Annulae.

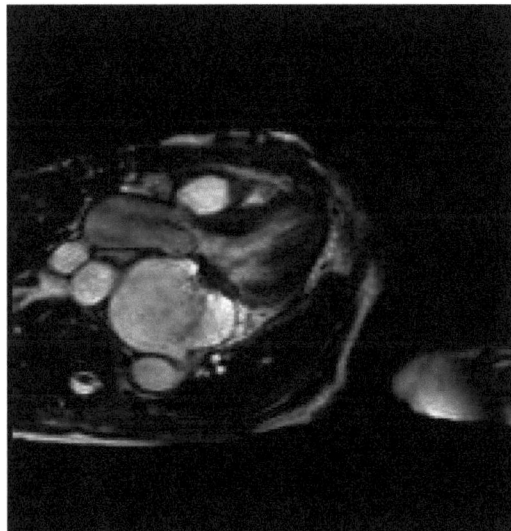

Figure 24b: Further Magnetic Resonance Imaging of the Same Patient but a Different Plane to Show the Aortic and Prosthetic Valve Annulae Relative Positions.

TAVI PROCEDURAL DETAILS

Pre-Operative Preparation

Once a patient has been fully assessed and accepted for TAVI the pre-operative preparation is not too dissimilar to a standard surgical approach. Anticoagulants should be stopped at least 5 days prior to the implant such that the INR is below 1.5. Oral anti-platelets should also be withheld as bleeding is one of the most important and prevalent complications. Haematological, biochemical and coagulation testing should be performed as well as cross matching two to four units of blood. An ECG should again be performed to reaffirm normal conduction, or otherwise. Pre-operative hydration is important for all patients, especially those with pre-existing renal impairment, as are prophylactic antibiotics according to local protocols. Patients with severe hepatic or renal disease may benefit from input from the appropriate specialists immediately pre-operative. All patients should have their chest and both groins (or radial puncture site) thoroughly cleaned and clipped.

TAVIs should only be performed with provisions for on-site surgery such that conversion to open procedure can occur immediately if required. The catheter suite should have high quality imaging as well as being equipped with a cardiopulmonary bypass machine (Fig. **25**), piped anaesthetics gases, vacuum and gas scavenging [20]. The concept of a hybrid catheter laboratory/operating theatre is ideal for such procedures [20, 21].

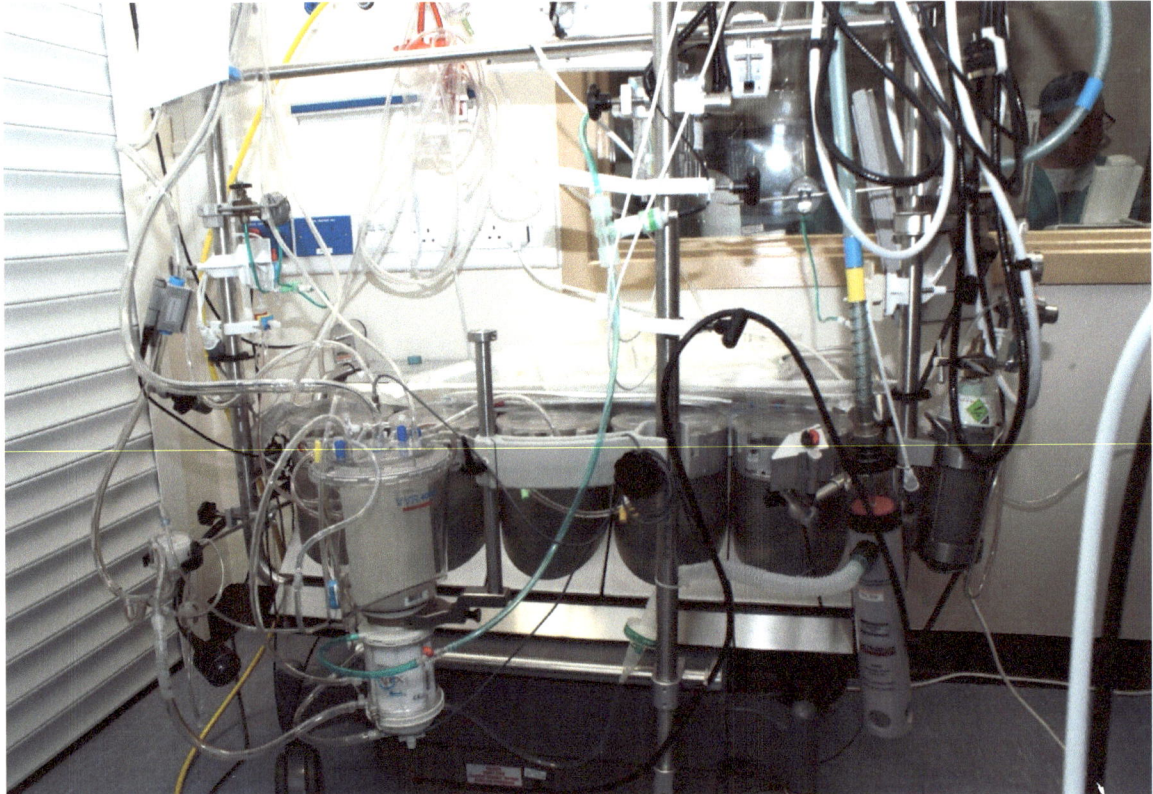

Figure 25: Cardiopulmonary Bypass Machine on Standby within the Corner of the Catheter Laboratory.

Immediate Pre-Implant Preparation

This will vary between cardiothoracic centres particularly as some centres do transfemoral procedures under local anaesthetic. There are preparatory steps which are common regardless of the implant approach. Large bore intravenous and arterial access should be acquired and a urinary catheter inserted. Central venous access can be acquired for pressure monitoring, fluid and drug administration. Patients should be continually warmed throughout the case, including fluid warming with close monitoring of the patients temperature.

For a transapical procedure the apex can be initially localised and marked using a transthoracic echo probe. Hands free defibrillator pads should be applied to the patient in a position where they would not interfere with any incision. After induction of anaesthesia the patient is prepared and draped.

Transoesophageal echocardiography (TOE) is performed to re-assess left ventricular function as well as aortic anatomy and physiology. The TOE probe will then remain in place for the duration of the procedure. Femoral venous and arterial sheaths are inserted. The arterial sheath allows delivery of a pigtail catheter to the aortic root. A trans-radial approach can be used in the event of peripheral access problems. The venous sheath enables a temporary pacing lead to be positioned in the right ventricular apex such that it can pace at low threshold. Any balloon device should only be expanded in the left ventricular outflow tract (LVOT) during high rate pacing. This should be tested such that the rate selected e.g. 180 beats per minute, drops the mean blood pressure to less than 40mmHg. This will stabilise equipment and prevent ejection from the LVOT during balloon inflation. Should ventricular fibrillation be precipitated at the time of valve deployment consider completing the implantation before defibrillating.

A critical preparatory step is finding a fluoroscopic angle whereby all the aortic sinuses are in absolute alignment (Fig. **26**). This is done by undertaking intermittent contrast injections though the pigtail catheter with slight adjustments to angulation of the X-ray camera. Once this angle has been found the operator can be confident of valve position relative to the annulus during positioning. This step is especially important for balloon mounted devices which are shorter from top to bottom making accurate placement essential. If the valve is deployed off axis it may miss one aortic leaflet completely, have inadequate support and potentially embolise.

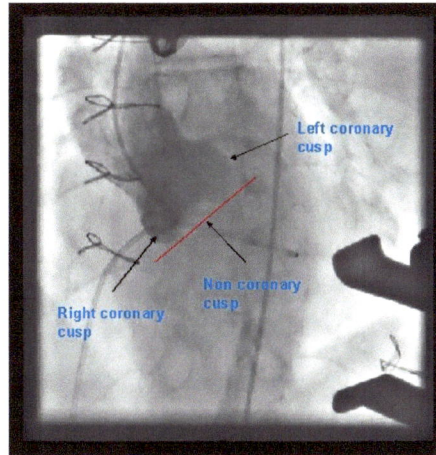

Figure 26: Adjust the Angulation of the X-Ray C-arm such that the Lowest Points of the Coronary Cusps are all in a Straight Line. This becomes the Working View for Valve Implantation.

Prior to any TAVI a balloon aortic valvuloplasty should be undertaken (in a similar manner to that described elsewhere) after appropriate upsizing of the femoral sheath or *via* the transapical introducer. An appropriately undersized balloon should be selected so as to avoid excessive native valve injury, for example a 20x30mm balloon. The midpoint is positioned at the annular level. The balloon is rapidly inflated and deflated during rapid pacing. A dilute concentration of contrast, such as 15%, should be used for this purpose to facilitate rapid filling and emptying of the balloon.

A single, stable yet full balloon inflation should be the target. If the balloon continually embolizes, either down into the ventricle or upwards in to the aorta the case may have to be stopped at this stage. Recurrent embolization may herald impending dislocation of the balloon mounted prosthesis. Balloon inflation also allows an opportunity to assess leaflet movement relative to the coronary ostia (See Figs. **27a** and **b**). If the leaflets move such that they could potentially occlude the coronaries during the TAVI it is unsafe to proceed further than a valvuloplasty. A test injection of contrast *via* the pigtail catheter at the time of maximal balloon inflation can be helpful in that regard.

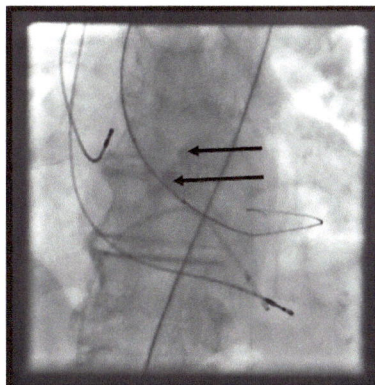

Figure 27a: The Arrows Indicate the Natural Position of the Thickened, Heavily Calcified Leaflets.

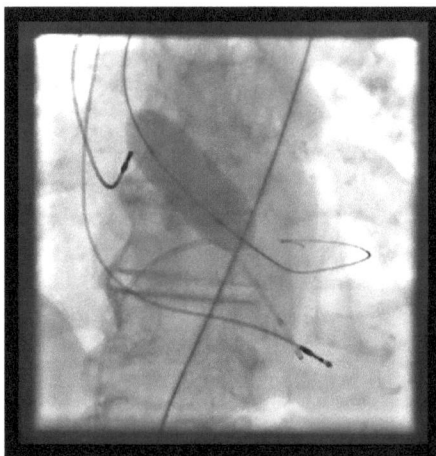

Figure 27b: With Balloon Inflation the Aortic Valve Leaflets can be Easily seen to Hinge Upwards, Potentially Occluding the Coronary Ostia should they be Low Lying.

It is a higher risk indicator if the blood pressure takes time to recover following cessation of high rate pacing. The hypotensive period should be as short as possible although giving sufficient time for the balloon to adequately deflate. Patients with poor left ventricular function and/or a large ischaemic burden are at increased risk from prolonged hypotension. Patients with labile blood pressure may require vasopressors or, under certain circumstances, cardiopulmonary bypass . Catecholamines should be avoided as they may worsen hypotension as should nitrous oxide on induction.

TRANSFEMORAL AORTIC VALVE IMPLANTATION

The appropriate leg for the large calibre delivery system would have been chosen following the evaluation process. To begin with centres usually choose to do a cut down procedure on to the femoral artery. This has a number of advantages. Firstly, it ensures that any calcified plaques can be avoided by direct vision thereby minimising injury and aiding vascular repair later. Secondly, a puncture into the larger calibre common femoral artery is more likely to be guaranteed. Thirdly, it avoids a puncture on to the side wall of the artery. Different methods of arterial exposure can be employed. Commonly the anterior wall of the artery is exposed leaving the posterior wall undissected for added support. The Seldinger needle then punctures through the skin below the incision, is passed into the operative field and through the anterior wall of the artery choosing the exact puncture site carefully. A 0.038/0.035 guide wire is then passed in to the iliac system, the needle removed and a 6 or 8F cannula introduced. *Via* the contra-lateral femoral artery the guiding pigtail catheter should be delivered to the ascending aorta. The corresponding femoral vein is a conduit to the right ventricular apex for a temporary pacing wire.

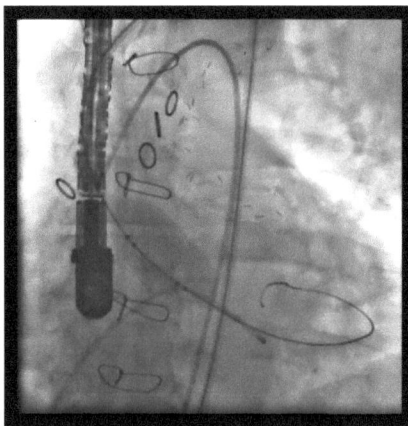

Figure 28: Initial Balloon Aortic Valvuloplasty. A Safe Loop of Wire can be Seen in the Left Ventricle to Minimize the Risk of Left Ventricular Perforation.

A 6F coronary catheter guided by a J tipped 0.035/0.038 wire is passed up to the aortic root. This catheter is then used to direct a straight wire retrogradely through the aortic valve orifice. The precise catheter used is at the discretion of the operator but could be an amplatz left 1 or 2, Judkins right 4, or a pigtail catheter. Upon crossing the valve with the straight wire the catheter is advanced carefully into the left ventricular cavity. An aortic valve gradient can be measured at this stage if desired. With the catheter within the left ventricle the straight wire is changed for an exchange length Amplatz super-stiff 0.035 guide-wire. Alternative guide-wires can be used if a stiffer or more relaxed delivery rail is required. It is usual to manually create a large loop on the ventricular end of the chosen wire to minimize the risk of left ventricular perforation. The wire left in-situ after catheter removal subsequently becomes the rail for aortic valve implantation.

Whilst keeping the wire safely in the ventricle the femoral sheath can be up-sized to facilitate delivery of the chosen aortic valvuloplasty balloon, usually at least 9F in calibre. Balloon aortic valvuloplasty (BAV) is performed (as described elsewhere) under high rate pacing (Fig. **29**). When a satisfactory stable, complete inflation has occurred preparations begin for the valve delivery.

The BAV introducer sheath is removed ensuring the wire remains safely within the left ventricle. The femoral artery is then dilated under fluoroscopic guidance using the accompanying hydrophilic dilators. The final size of the introducer sheath is determined by the desired valve size (check manufacturers instructions). After safe dilatation the final introducer catheter is placed into the iliofemoral artery under screening such that it is coaxial to the aorta. The introducer sheath should be secured either by a suture or by assistance to avoid tip movement and migration injuring the aortic wall. It is also recommended the sheath be gently rotated every few minutes to prevent adhesion of the hydrophilic coating to the endothelium of the iliac artery.

During this time a separate team of assistants would have been preparing and crimping the appropriately sized aortic prosthetic valve on to the delivery system (Fig. **30**). The team should ensure there is minimal delay in completing the case after the BAV particularly if severe aortic valve regurgitation has ensued in the context of poor left ventricular function. The orientation of the prosthetic unidirectional valve has to be checked by the principle operator prior to it passing in to the introducer. The crimped valve and delivery catheter can then be advanced over the guide wire in to the aortic lumen under fluoroscopic guidance. For balloon mounted systems this is the point of no return, the prosthesis, even if not deployed can only be removed surgically from here on.

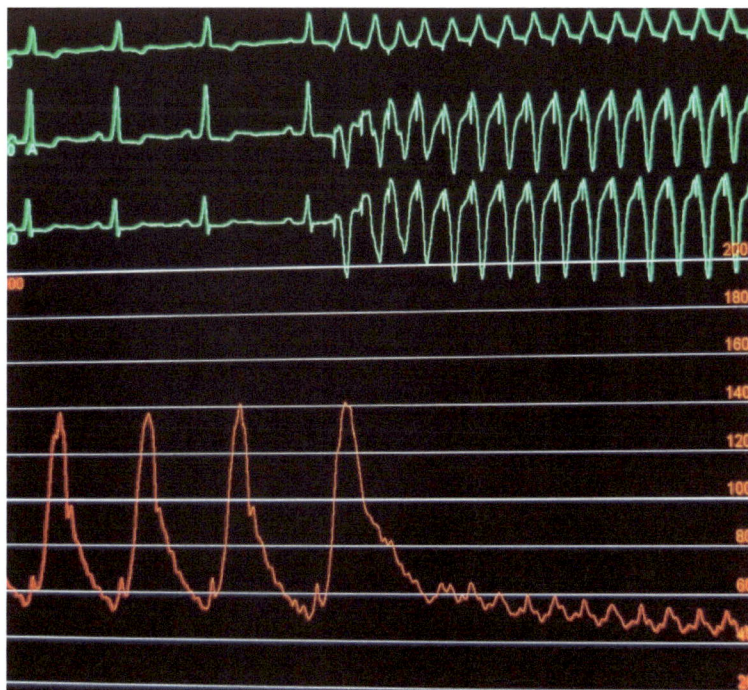

Figure 29: High Rate Pacing.

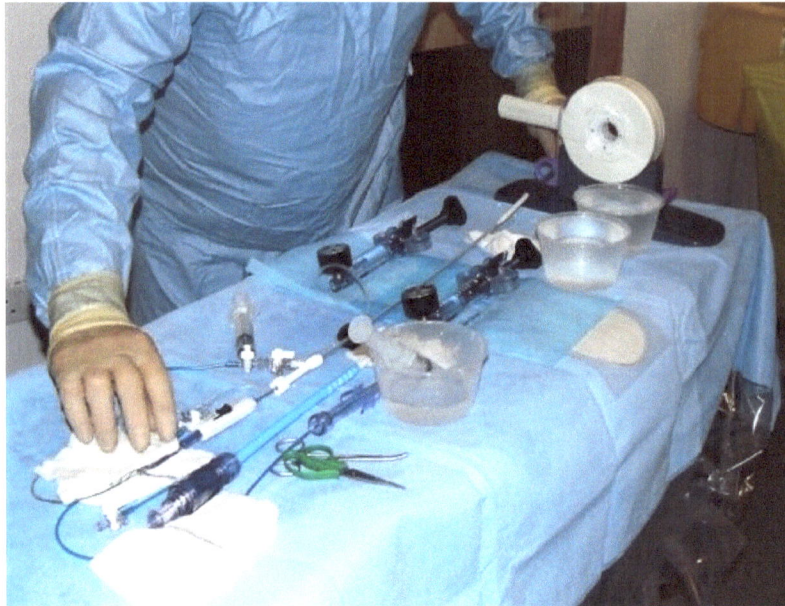

Figure 30: Independent Preparation of the Valvuloplasty Balloon, Prosthetic Valve, and the Steerable Delivery. The Crimping Device can be seen at the Far End of the Sterile Table.

The steering mechanism should direct the crimped valve around the aortic arch to the root. The steerability can also be used to subsequently cross and find a coaxial, central position within the native valve. Throughout all these steps it is important that the external end of the wire is anchored by an assistant and that care is taken not to force too much wire in to the ventricle risking perforation. Once retrogradely across the valve it is very important to retract the "pusher" component of the delivery system such that it will not interfere with the impending balloon inflation.

Valve positioning is optimised in the working view using fluoroscopic imaging and intermittent contrast injections *via* the pigtail (Fig. **31**). It can be useful to push the pigtail deeply into the aortic sinus to indicate the lowest point of the leaflet. Usually the other leaflets can be visualised by the calcification. Due to force of ventricular ejection a slight cranial displacement of the valve should be expected. A position biased towards the ventricle, for example *i.e.* 2/3rds of the prosthesis in the ventricle, $1/3^{rd}$ in the valve, will account for this movement. Transoesophageal echocardiography will become increasingly important for positioning especially with the increasing availability of real time 3D imaging systems. The final position is checked prior to deployment during rapid pacing often with ventilation transiently suspended.

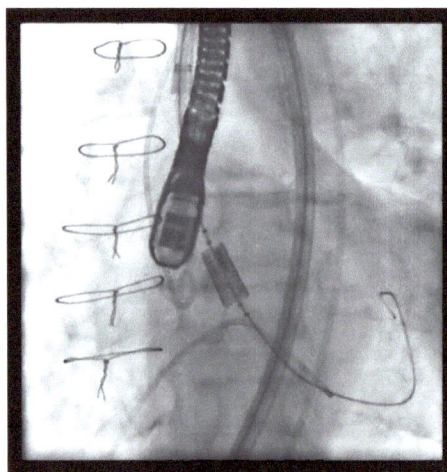

Figure 31: With the Prosthesis within the Native Aortic Valve the Retroflex Catheter and the Pusher should be Retracted to Fully Expose the Balloon and to Allow Final Positioning.

When the team is satisfied that the prosthesis is optimally positioned it is ready for deployment. Balloon mounted valves are deployed in the manner of a BAV by maximally inflating and deflating the balloon under direct pacing (Fig. **32**). It is important to wait for the mean blood pressure to trough before inflation and then for the balloon to maximally deflate before the pacing stops to avoid ventricular systole ejection the apparatus in the outflow tract. The balloon should then be withdrawn back in to the ascending aorta to allow the new prosthesis to function (Fig. **33**).

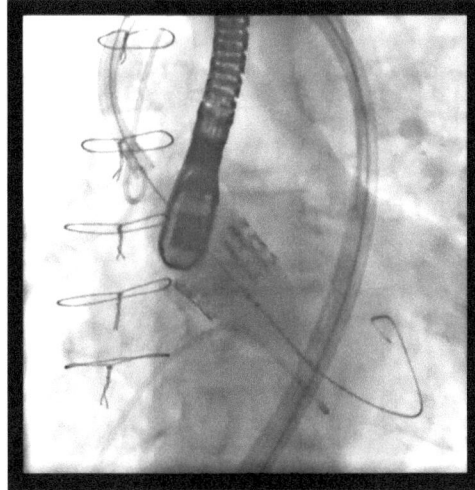

Figure 32: Balloon Inflation During High Rate Pacing with Expansion and Subsequent Deployment of the Valve.

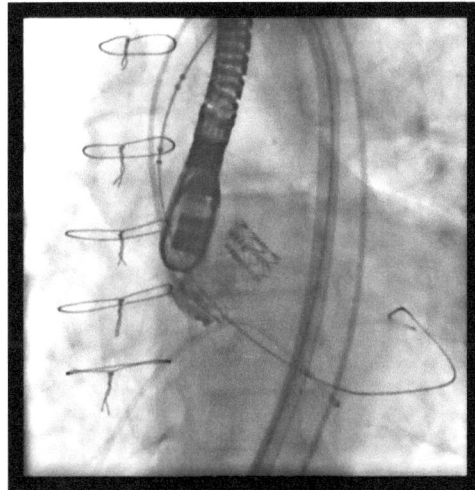

Figure 33: Fully Deployed Edward Sapien Valve Undergoing Assessment by Transoesophageal Echocardiography Prior to Removal of the Wire.

Following successful deployment the prosthesis is checked for valvular and paravalvular regurgitation by using principally TOE but also contrast aortography. With the wire still across valvular regurgitation is expected. Time is also required for the leaflets to reach body temperature and become compliant. If significant paraprosthetic regurgitation is seen a further balloon dilatation may be required. This is done in perhaps 25% of cases. Further ballooning does carry risk of valve embolization as well as valve injury. If severe valvular regurgitation is seen then a second prosthesis may be required inside the first. Final checks for aortic regurgitation are then made once the wire has been removed.

Upon completion of valve implantation the steerable catheter is fully released and removed. The introducer is then also removed and checks made to exclude vascular injury before surgical repair of the arteriotomy or the application of a closure device.

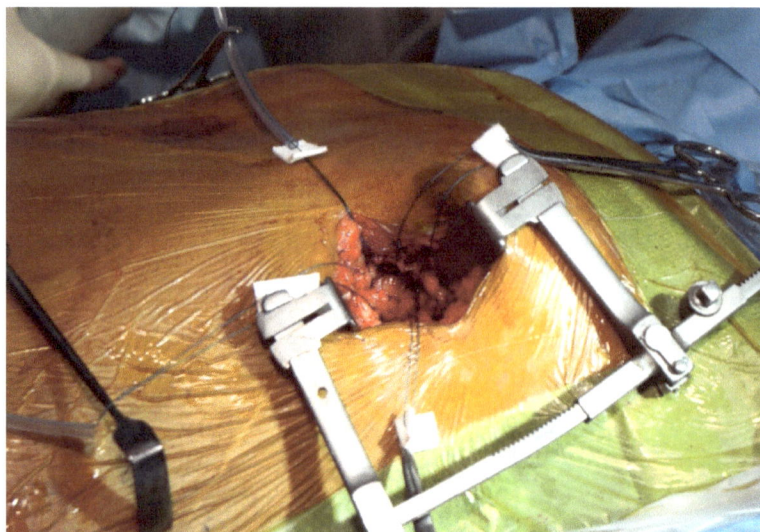

Figure 34: Transapical Surgical Field with Rib Retractors and Pledgeted Sutures in Place. The Ventricle is Ready for Puncture with the Seldinger Needle.

If there have been no concerns regarding atrio-ventricular conduction the right ventricular pacing lead can be removed immediately. Alternatively it can be left in as required. The contra-lateral arterial sheath can be removed immediately. The patient is recovered and then transferred to an intensive care unit, a high dependency unit or the ward as appropriate.

COREVALVE IMPLANTATION

The Corevalve Revalving system consists of a self expanding prosthesis. Vascular access can again be achieved by cut down or percutaneous puncture of the common femoral, common iliac or subclavian arteries depending upon the suitability of the vasculature for the delivery of device. Balloon aortic valvuloplasty is again performed with high rate pacing as described elsewhere before the device deployment. A 0.035 Amplatz wire is placed in the left ventricle over which the delivery system is railed. The device is positioned across the native valve and correct position is adjusted with the help of fluoroscopy using the calcified aortic leaflets as an anatomical marker as well transoesophageal echocardiogram. The sheath is pulled back which leads to the delivery of the self expandable prosthetic valve.

A self expanding system does have a number of advantages. High rate pacing for deployment is not mandated. The implant time can, therefore be much longer as hypotension is avoided. The device can also be repositioned, and even recovered completely, if necessary should there be difficulty with deployment.

Finally, an aortogram and TOE are performed to confirm successful deployment of the valve and to assess the degree of aortic regurgitation and whether any further intervention is required.

TRANSAPICAL AORTIC VALVE IMPLANTATION

This technique is most applicable for patients with small, diseased or tortuous peripheral vessels or issues with the aorta. It follows the same general principle of a transfemoral approach but as the distance from the native aortic valve to the operator is a relatively short, straight line valve delivery tends to be technically a more stable procedure.

Prior to draping and making the final operative preparations the apex, and the appropriate rib space through which to access the left ventricle, is identified by palpation and echocardiography. A mini thoracotomy is subsequently undertaken with rib retraction and dissection down and through the parietal pericardium. An appropriate puncture position of the apex or anterior ventricular wall is chosen by direct inspection. Pledgeted sutures are placed in the myocardium around the proposed access point (Fig. **34**). This encircled area is punctured with a Seldinger needle through which is passed a 0.035 J tip standard guide wire. The wire often passes easily through the left ventricular outflow tract and antegradely across the aortic valve, around the aortic arch to the descending aorta. Care should be taken to avoid a route through the submitral apparatus. This may only become apparent as subsequent larger calibre equipment is delivered and may lead to procedural failure. The needle is then removed and a coronary catheter, for example Judkins right 4, passed to the descending aorta over the wire which is then removed. A 180cm amplatz extra stiff 0.035 wire is delivered to the descending aorta. The operators should again be vigilant about proximal or distal migration of the wire tip. The coronary catheter is exchanged for the BAV introducer sheath or directly to the transapical valve introducer (Ascendra). The myocardial puncture site does not require graded dilatation. Transfemoral arterial and venous sheaths can be used for the guiding aortic root pigtail and right ventricular pacing lead. Alternatively epicardial pacing leads can be used for the purpose of high rate pacing during balloon inflation.

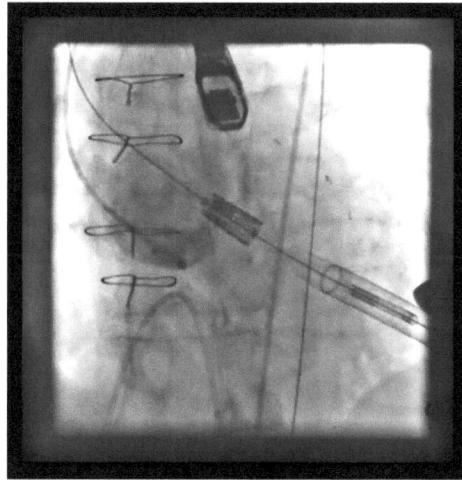

Figure 35: Positioning of the Prosthetic Valve within the Stenotic Aortic Valve *via* the Transapical Delivery System.

A 20mm aortic valvuloplasty balloon is invariably utilised to perform BAV under high rate pacing. After achieving a stable aortic valvuloplasty with full balloon inflation without evidence of coronary compromise one can proceed to TAVI. The BAV balloon is removed and the appropriate calibre introducer placed though the apex over the wire ensuring it does not cross, and potentially occlude, the aortic valve orifice.

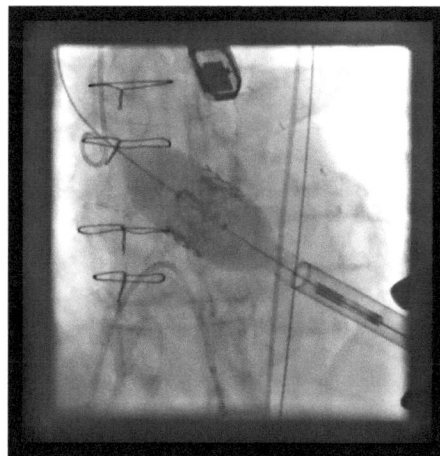

Figure 36: Final Deployment of a Balloon Expandable Valve Delivered *via* the Transapical Route.

The transapical balloon mounted prosthesis is prepared and positioned in a similar manner to a transfemoral approach but with very important differences (Fig. **35**). Firstly, and most importantly, it must be ensured that the unidirectional valve is correctly oriented on the balloon such that it is suitable for an antegrade approach. Secondly, the delivery system is much shorter and straighter than transfemoral equipment. As a result balloons are more stable with less cranial drift during inflation. Therefore, on positioning just 50% of the valve should be in the ventricle, 50% within the native leaflets to hopefully deploy in the perfect position within the aortic valve annulus. The operator must again ensure the pusher is fully retracted such that it does not squeeze the balloon forward with inflation leading to valve embolization.

Final deployment of the valve is essentially identical to the delivery of a transfemoral balloon mounted prosthesis (Fig. **36**); use the working fluoroscopic view combined with echocardiography, high rate pacing with ventilation suspended, rapid balloon inflation and deflation, pull back the balloon to allow the valve to function, assess once more with echocardiography and fluoroscopy making any further interventions as appropriate (Fig. **37**).

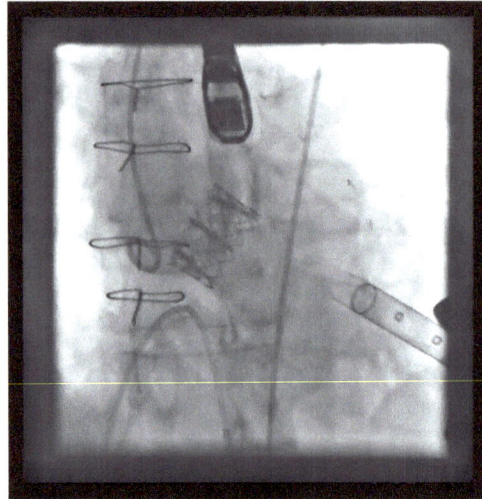

Figure 37: Final Result of the Fully Deployed Valve with no Evidence of Aortic Regurgitation.

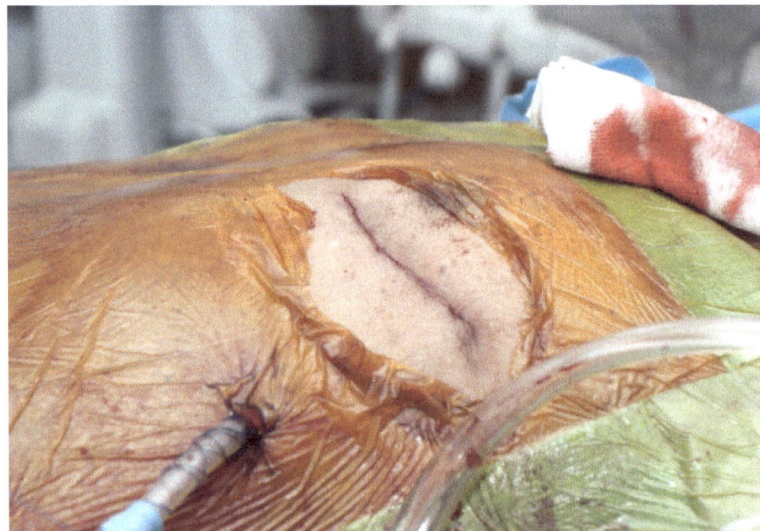

Figure 38: Following Final Closure of the Transapical Wound with One Drain Left in-situ.

Once the team is satisfied the valve is well positioned and performing optimally the balloon tip is placed back carefully across the valve such that the distal marker is just above the level of the prosthesis. The wire can then be safely retracting avoiding valve injury. The whole apparatus is then removed from the apex and haemostasis achieved using the previously placed pledgeted sutures. The pericardium is approximated with a drain in-situ and the wound closed (Fig. **38**). Protamine can be given at this stage to reverse the heparin. Intercostal nerve blocks can be used for post-operative analgesia. The femoral/radial arterial sheath can be removed before the patient leaves the catheter laboratory.

POST IMPLANT CARE

Tracheal extubation can often take place at the end of the procedure. Close post-operative monitoring is required hence patients are transferred to either a specific recovery area or the intensive care unit. Once stable and recovered patients can either remain in intensive care or be transferred to a high dependency unit or cardiothoracic ward depending on the specific circumstances. This transfer can be within a few hours for selected patients. Transapical wounds can be painful hence the use of local nerve blocks and patient controlled analgesia. Transfemoral patients tend to recover faster as they are less restricted by pain.

If there are no concerns regarding intraventricular conduction the pacing leads can be removed immediately after the procedure or later as directed by the operators. If irreversible conduction block has occurred the pacing leads should remain until the permanent pacemaker is implanted.

If there are no haemorrhagic concerns the patient should have loading doses of aspirin and clopidogrel as soon as practically possible. Dual antiplatelet therapy is continued for a minimum of 3 months with aspirin continuing for life.

Patients can be mobilised from day 1 with the aim of a total hospital stay between 3 and 7 days. The duration is likely to shorten with increasing experience and smaller calibre equipment. A predischarge baseline echocardiogram is advisable which can be repeated at 3, 6, and 12 months.

COMPLICATIONS OF TRANSCATHETER AORTIC IMPLANTATION

The same general complications which can occur after cardiac surgery (infection, bleeding) or any other transcatheter intervention (contrast nephropathy, false aneurysm formation) can occur after TAVI but there are some which are specific to these procedures and merit discussion.

1. Device Embolization

For balloon mounted devices this occurs largely due to the systolic force of left ventricular contraction pushing the inflated balloon, and hence prosthesis, out of the left ventricular outflow tract. The risk for this is dramatically reduced by rapid pacing which offloads the ventricle and reduces the mean blood pressure. It is important to ensure that pacing is not stopped prematurely and that there is no failure to capture during device deployment.

Embolization may also be secondary to anatomical balloon migration. This could be due to prominent bulging of the basal septum or a mitral valve prosthesis. The potential for device embolization in these scenarios can be assessed during the BAV phase of the procedure. If the balloon recurrently embolizes it would be recommended that the case finish at that point rather than risk device embolization. A transapical procedure may be more applicable for these cases as there is inherently less balloon drift on inflation. The operator is also able to apply some counter traction due to the shorter system.

It is unusual for the device to embolize into the ventricle. This usually occurs because the attempted deployment position was too low in the first place. This is best avoided by taking care to find the very best perpendicular working view and taking the time to find the optimal valve position using fluoroscopy, aortography and transoesophageal echocardiography.

Once the prosthesis has left the introducer it can only be removed surgically. Therefore, if the device displaces cranially the best strategy is to manipulate it around the aortic arch and deploy it in the descending thoracic aorta. It is extremely important not to lose wire position as the valve will immediately turn over due to blood flow and coapt. In this event the operators should try and recross and potentially stent it open. A further TAVI device can then be placed in to the aortic valve annulus to complete the case.

An embolization in to the ventricle is harder to deal with and may mandate a conversion to open sternotomy. In a transapical procedure it may be possible to hook the prosthesis and suture it to the inside of the ventricle in a compressed position. Sometimes the valve prosthesis may be insecure within the aortic annulus but not free. In these circumstances a second device can be placed inside the first such as to stabilise its position. For all of these reasons it is advisable to have ready access to a cardiopulmonary bypass machine and spare valves.

2. Aortic Regurgitation

Mild to moderate aortic regurgitation is often very well tolerated and is a reasonable trade off for critical aortic valve stenosis. Acute severe aortic regurgitation may not be well tolerated in a hypertrophied noncompliant left ventricle or a poorly functioning ventricle with or without significant areas of ischaemia. Valvular regurgitation after TAVI can only be properly assessed after removal of the wire as it will inevitably restrict valvular function. It is normal to have a mild degree of regurgitation initially until the leaflets have achieved full flexibility at body temperature. Severe regurgitation may occur because of leaflet failure or because of poor deployment. A second valve may thus be required. Occasionally the prosthetic leaflets may be tethered or everted in which case very gentle probing may be helpful.

Paraprosthetic regurgitation has a number of potential mechanisms. A secondary intervention should only be undertaken if the degree of leak is moderate or greater. Any further balloon dilatation carries the risk of injuring the leaflets or promoting device embolization. The valve may simply be under expanded in which case it should be helped by further balloon expansion. Undersizing of the valve should have been avoided by careful pre-operative measurement of the aortic valve annulus.

The native valve disease leads to nodular calcific degeneration. A paraprosthetic leak occurs in some patients if the calcification is very eccentric. Again this may respond to further dilatation. Often paraprosthetic regurgitation can improve spontaneously over time as the native valve organises around the stent frame essentially plugging the gaps. Very severe leaks can potentially be treated by endovascular devices. TAVI prostheses are designed such that the lower portion is covered with fabric. If the prosthesis is too low regurgitation in to the ventricle can occur above the level the fabric in which case a second device, placed slightly higher, yet still within the first device may be indicated.

3. Coronary Occlusion

These procedures are not valve replacements but implantations. As such the native leaflets remain in situ and are pushed aside by the prosthesis. There is, therefore, a risk of occluding the coronary ostia as the valve leaflets hinge upwards during device placement. Patients with low lying coronary ostia are at particular risk and they should be screened out during assessment. If there is concern of potential coronary compromise during the TAVI it is recommended that a contrast injection be performed during BAV to assess the relative relation of the leaflet tips and the coronaries. If the coronaries are seen to be covered by the leaflets the procedure should be stopped at that point. Emergency angioplasty or a conversion to open surgery could be performed if the coronaries are inadvertently occluded by the native valve leaflets during prosthetic placement.

4. Vascular Complications

These are the most common complications of Transfemoral procedures. Dissection and perforation of the peripheral vasculature have all been reported, either the aorta or iliofemoral vessels. It is advisable that equipment, such as aortic occlusion balloons, covered stents, balloon expandable stents, etc., are available to repair any peripheral problems that may occur. All iliofemoral arteries should be carefully inspected by angiography for any potential injury before the patient leaves the catheter laboratory. Some cases may require involvement of vascular surgeons and/or interventional radiologists before, during and after the procedure.

CLINICAL EVIDENCE

Aortic balloon valvuloplasty provides symptomatic relief but does not benefit mortality [3, 22-26]. BAV is, therefore, a palliative therapy in severely symptomatic patients or a bridge to definitive surgery for certain select unstable patients [20]. No randomised study data is yet available comparing TAVI to either medical therapy or high risk surgery. Results from PARTNER-US trial should be available in late 2010. The aim is to enrol 1048 patients with randomisation to a surgical arm comparing the Edward sapien valve with open valve surgery and medical arm comparing transcatheter valve replacement with medical therapy and balloon valvuloplasty in patients considered too high risk for conventional surgery. The primary end point is death at 1 year while secondary points include a composite cardiovascular event, valve performance and quality of life.

ANTEGRADE TRANSVENOUS APPROACH

The first device was implanted in 2002 by Cribier [2]. The early procedures were undertaken on a compassionate basis in patients with NYHA class IV symptoms with an equine trileaflet valve. The reports from that time demonstrated feasibility of the concept but the results were difficult to reproduce and the operative mortality risk was 25 % [14]. The early registries of I-REVIVE and RECAST reported successful implantation in 27 out of 36 high risk patients [8, 14, 27]. There was improvement in symptoms, valve area and gradient overall, although 5 patients had significant aortic regurgitation (grade 3) Major adverse effects cardiovascular events occurred in seven patients (26%) at 30 days and in another 10 patients in the next six months. Ultimately 10 patients were followed up for at least one year, 4 for at least 2 years and 2 for at least 3 years [27, 28].

The technical complexity of transvenous approach, led to the development of the retrograde transfemoral technique.

TRANSARTERIAL APPROACH

This is now the method of choice for TAVI if technically possible. Webb *et al [*3]. reported single centre results in the pioneering first 50 high risk patients with a retrograde implantation of the original Cribier equine balloon expandable valve. High risk status was adjudicated by consensus of a multidisciplinary team of surgeons and cardiologists when conventional surgical risk was considered excessive. The mean logistic EuroSCORE was 28 with a mean age of 82 years. Intraprocedural mortality was 2% with a procedural success overall of 86%. This was lower in the first 25 patients, 76%, but much higher in the second consecutive cohort of 25 patients, improving to 96%. This reflected the learning curve combined with technological development. Reasons for failure included an inability to cross the valve in 3 patients, unsuitable iliacs in 1 patient and malpositioning in 2 patients. In both of the latter cases, the prosthesis became free in the ascending aorta. The valves were withdrawn with the delivery catheter and further dilated and fixed within the transverse aorta in a location where major branch vessels would not be compromised. One patient some time later underwent elective conventional AVR at 103 days. The second patient continues on medical management for aortic stenosis. The perioperative stroke rate was 4% [30, 31, 32, 33].

Mean gradient dropped from 46 +/-17 to 11+/-5 mmHg with an increase in valve area from 0.6 +/-0.2 to 1.7+/-0.4cm2. Moderate paravalvular regurgitation was seen in 3 patients. The haemodynamic improvement was reflected in the symptoms, with most patients jumping at least one functional class, as well as improved LV function and mitral regurgitation. Within 30 days 12% of patients died; related to left main occlusion, stroke, iliac artery perforation, multi-system failure and malignant arrhythmias. The 30 day mortality was again lower for the second cohort of 25 patients relative to the first; 16% to 8%. No patient required open heart surgery within this early period. At one year 81% of the patients who underwent successful valve implant were alive with echocardiography confirming persistent structural integrity of the valve. The early improvement in symptoms continued to be observed at 6 and 12 months.

A small early French study reports the outcome of 12 patients undergoing valve implantation with a predicted operative risk >20% [30]. They were mostly in NYHA class IV (75%) with a mean age of 85 years. In-hospital mortality was high at 25% but there were no additional deaths by six months. The mean functional class of survivors by this stage was 2.

The multicentre Canadian experience allows assessment of a larger cohort of patients treated by the transarterial approach [34]. A Tran femoral implant was attempted in 167 patients, although failed in 6 (ultimately treated transapically) mostly due to failure of iliofemoral navigation. Mean age was 83 years, 92.6% were in NYHA class III or IV, with a mean aortic gradient of 48 mmHg and LV ejection fraction of 55%. Procedural mortality was 1.8% with a 2% rate of conversion to open surgery. There were 5 occasions (3%) of valve embolisation requiring a second valve in 4 instances. The rate of stroke and coronary obstruction were both 0.6%. Thirty day mortality was 9.5% and a pacemaker requirement of 3.6%. As the paper reports combined results for transapical and transfemoral approaches it is not possible to extract detailed information specific to the transarterial approach.

The largest registry to date is the SOURCE registry of the Edwards valve [35]. All patients undergoing a TAVI within the first year of commercial availability in 32 spearheading centres were included. Transfemoral patients made up just half of the total patient sample, 463 out of 1038. The average age was 81.7 years with a EuroSCORE of 25.7%, a score greater than 20 in 70%. Acute procedural success occurred in 95.6%. Surgical conversion was required in 1.7% with a 0.7% incidence of coronary occlusion. Thirty day survival was 93.7% continuing the steady improvement observed through previous studies. The 30 day stroke rate was 2.4%, pacemaker requirement rate of 6.7% and a dialysis rate of 5%. The biggest complication was again vascular injury with an incidence of 17.9% but unlike previous studies it was no longer a predictor of procedural mortality.

The first reported CoreValve series was in 2006 [8]. Patients all had severe aortic valve stenosis and were felt to be at prohibitive surgical risk. Arterial access was gained either through the subclavian, common iliac or common femoral artery by surgical cutdown. Cardiopulmonary bypass was used for all patients. The patients were mostly females with a mean age just over 80 years. NYHA III or IV was present in 96% with a median EuroSCORE of 11.0%. Acute procedural success was 84%, emergency surgery being required in 2 patients. The in-hospital mortality rate was 1 in 5. The same clinical group later showed feasibility and successful haemodynamic and symptomatic improvement with both the first generation and subsequent second generation device [31, 33].

A larger German/Canadian study (n=86) reported the use of the second and third generation CoreValve *via* retrograde transvascular methods [9]. Patients again had severe aortic valve stenosis with different EuroSCORE criteria depending on the age. The mean age was 82.2 years, with 65% being female, a mean EuroSCORE of 21.7 and mean peak gradient of 70.9mmHg. Adequate device insertion was obtained in 88% of the cohort. In 6 patients, misplacement of the valve led to urgent conversion to operative valve replacement. In 2 patients, the device did not cross the heavily calcified native valve despite a balloon predilatation. In a further 2 patients, a suboptimal placement of the prosthesis with remaining aortic regurgitation had to be corrected by implantation of a second CoreValve prosthesis (prosthesis-in-prosthesis).The overall procedural success rate was reported as 74%. The overall procedural MACCE rate excluding patients with conversion to valvuloplasty or surgery was 18%. Five deaths occurred periprocedurally: 2 patients died after conversion to balloon valvuloplasty and surgical aortic valve replacement 3 patients died of pericardial tamponade. Overall tamponade occurred in 9 patients: 6 were likely caused by wire perforations of the ventricle. Two cases occurred in the postoperative phase after urgent conversion to operative valve replacement. One case complicated pacemaker implantation. No coronary obstruction was observed in the series but the stroke rate was high at 10%.

Overall 30 day mortality was 12%. In patients with device and procedural success, the mortality was 9% and 5%, respectively. Significant improvements in functional class were again noted from NYHA 2.85 beforehand to 1.85 afterwards. Worsening aortic regurgitation relative to baseline occurred in 26 patients due to paravalvular leak but no patients had a severe grade. Stroke occurred in 10% and cardiac tamponade in 9% of the group.

A different group has reported outcomes on thirty patients with severe aortic valve stenosis and a contraindication to surgery treated with the third generation device [36]. Mean age was 82 years with an average peak gradient of 85.6mmHg, valve area of 0.61cm, ejection fraction of 52.6% and a EuroSCORE of 25.3%. Acute device success was achieved in 97%. One patient required a second CoreValve because of malposition of the first. One patient had a non-fatal tamponade. New onset complete heart block requiring a permanent pacemaker occurred in 20%. The 30 day mortality was 6.7% with 2 patients dying after suffering a stroke. Mean NYHA functional class declined from 2.7 pre-procedure to 1.31 afterwards.

A larger study reports 168 consecutive patients from 2 centres in receipt of a CoreValve from 2005 to 2008 [37]. Some of these patients would undoubtedly have been presented in former publications. The mean age was 81 years with 93% of patients in NYHA III/IV and a mean valve area of 0.66cm. The acute and in-hospital procedural success rates were 90.5 and 83.9%, respectively. The in-hospital MACCE rate was 16.7%, with an in-hospital mortality, myocardial infarction, and stroke rate of 11.9, 1.8, and 3.6%, respectively. In-hospital mortality was primarily related to progressive heart failure, dominantly right heart failure, as well as pneumonia, sepsis, and mesenteric infarction. Acute device success was observed in 93.5%.

Laborde has presented the European multicentre registry of CoreValve following the commercial launch of the 18F system [38]. Procedural success in 1243 patients had now to 98% with a near 50% reduction in implant times as well as reduced complication rates. Thirty day mortality is now reported to be 6.7% with a stroke rate of 1.4%.

Pacemaker rates seem to be lower at 12% than the earlier registries. The same registry now has data available for 1483 patients with slightly increased success rates and lower rates of mortality once more highlighting the learning curve effect [39].

TRANSAPICAL APPROACH.

The earliest report of a transapical approach came from the pioneering Vancouver group [2, 12]. The original 26mm Cribier Equine valve was implanted in 7 patients who had been refused surgery for severe aortic valve stenosis and were not suitable for a transiliofemoral approach. Excellent haemodynamic and echardiographic results were achieved. There was a single 30 day mortality due to pneumonia and 2 further deaths by six months [40, 41].

A larger series using the same technique and prosthesis was later published by the Leipzig group [42]. The cohort consisted of 30 patients, mean Euroscore of 11.3 +/- 1.7%, all with severely symptomatic aortic valve stenosis. Peripheral cardiopulmonary bypass was used on 13 occasions with an overall implant success in 29 of 30 patients. Three patients died in hospital and two required a permanent pacemaker. The same group later published results on the first 50 patients [16]. By then the mean EuroSCORE and age were higher. The valve implantation success rate was preserved although 3 patients required conversion to conventional surgery due to valve dislocation, aortic root dissection and coronary occlusion. Seven patients required renal dialysis, 3 of which had pre-existent renal disease. The 30 day mortality was 8% although by 12 months 29%. Mortality was stated to be non-valve related in all patients. The Leipzig group have now published ongoing results for 100 high risk aortic stenotic patients treated with the Edwards system [43]. There were no further reports of failure to implant no the valve or conversion to open surgery. The thirty day mortality was 10% and by 12 months 27%. None of the deaths were related to valve malfunction. There was no incidence of stroke but a 10.1% incidence or requiring a new pacemaker for high degree heart block. Excellent functional improvement was also demonstrated with all but seven patients improving by at least one NYHA functional class.

The Vancouver group also went on to publish their extended early series of 55 transapical patients [32]. The overall 30 day mortality rate was reported as 18.2%. Again the rate was higher at 25% in the first half of the cohort decreasing to 11.1% in the second half. In 2010 the 3 year results have been published representing the longest follow-up of transapical aortic valve implantation in humans [44]. Seventy one patients, all with severe symptomatic aortic valve stenosis and declined surgical intervention underwent valve implantation. The mean follow-up was 12.9 +/- 11.5 months (total of 917.3 months), mean age was 80.0years and mean predicted operative mortality by logistic EuroSCORE was 34.5% +/- 20.4%Valve implantation was successful in all patients. Thirty day mortality was 16.9% in all patients but 33% in the first 15 patients falling to 12.5% in the remainder. Ten died subsequently to give an overall survival at 24 and 36 months of 66.3% +/- 6.4% and 58.0% +/- 9.5%, respectively. Among 59 patients who survived at least 30 days, 24- and 36-month survivals were 79.8% +/- 6.4% and 69.8% +/- 10.9%, respectively. NYHA class improved significantly from a mean preoperatively of 3.3 to 1.8 at 24 months. The aortic valve area and mean gradient remained stable at 24 months. They conclude that transapical TAVI provides sustained clinical and haemodynamic benefits for up to 36 months.

A multicentre registry of the transapical approach was published in 2007 [16]. This included 56 patients from 4 centres in Europe and the United States. Average EuroScore was 11.2 +/-1.8 with a successful valve implant in 55 patients. Peripheral cardiopulmonary bypass was used in a in 28 patients overall and four required an early sternotomy. The in-hospital mortality was 13.6% with an actuarial survival of 75.7 +/-5.9% at a mean follow-up of 110+/-77 days. This was followed by a solely American study of feasibility of the Transapical technique in 40 patients [41]. Subjects were all over 70 years of age, severely symptomatic from aortic valve stenosis and tuned down for surgery or deemed to be at very high risk of complications. The EuroScore was high at 35% with a mean age of 83.0+/- 7.5. Success was achieved in 35 but sternotomy was required for 5 patients. There were 3 operative deaths, which had increased to 7 by day 30. In-hospital death totalled 9 patients. By 6 months the actuarial survival was 58.7% but this had been the highest risk population reported up to this point.

The largest multicentre registry of the Transapical technique has been recently published [45]. The SOURCE registry collected data of patients treated at European centres following the commercial release of the Edwards Sapien valve. Over a 12 month period 575 procedures were performed in 32 centres. Mean age was 80.7 years, mean

EuroScore 29.1% (40.9% had a EuroSCORE of 30 or greater) with 27.1% of patients having had prior surgery. Successful valve deployment (valve positioned, catheter retrieved, no conversion to surgery and the patient left the intervention room alive) took place in 92.7% with 3.5% requiring conversion to an open procedure. Coronary obstruction occurred in 0.7% and valve embolisation in 0.5%. The immediate post-implant degree of aortic regurgitation in excess of 2+ was present in 2.3%. Nineteen patients required a double "valve in valve" procedure for the correction of severe paravalvular regurgitation of valve malposition.

Total 30 day mortality in the SOURCE registry was 10.3%. A quarter of the patients that died did so within the first 72 hours. Heart failure and access related problems were the main causes of early death. Overall the majority of deaths were caused by multiorgan and heart failure (47.5%). A pacemaker was required in 7.3%, the stroke rate was 2.6% with a surprisingly high rate of dialysis at 7.1%; one third of patients had baseline renal dysfunction. The authors concluded that despite the complexity of TAVI, virginal programs could be started with appropriate training leading to the acquisition of favourable results particularly when considering the high risk profile of the patients treated. The SOURCE registry will later publish the 2 year outcome data of the first cohort as well the same measures for the second year of commercialisation.

CONCLUSION

Surgery remains the gold standard treatment for patients with symptomatic severe aortic valve stenosis. The novel transcatheter aortic valve techniques, however, represent a new paradigm opening up the prospect of aortic valve intervention to a wider population. With increasing trial data it is expected that TAVI indications will gradually increase, expanding for example into therapy for aortic valve regurgitation. Studies published to date have shown a consistent improvement in procedural success, a reduction in complications and an increase in survival whilst maintaining an excellent symptomatic response. As longer term in-vivo durability is demonstrated it would also be expected that TAVI becomes more applicable to lower risk populations at a younger age. Some clinicians would advocate a time when TAVI is the treatment of choice for any patient who does not require concomitant mandated coronary bypass grafting. Continued technological development will allow all procedures to get easier and safer with time whilst preserving results.

REFERENCES

[1]   Nkomo VT, Gardin JM, Skelton TN, Gottdiener JS, *et al.* Burden of valvular heart diseases: a population-based study. Lancet 2006; 368: 1005-1011.

[2]   Cribier A, Eltchaninoff H, Bash A, *et al.* Percutaneous transcatheter implantation of an aortic valve prosthesis for calcific aortic stenosis: first human case description Circulation 2002; 106: 3006-3008.

[3]   Webb JG, Chandavimol M, Thompson CR, *et al.* Percutaneous aortic valve implantation retrograde from the femoral artery. Circulation 2006; 113: 842-850.

[4]   Grube E, Laborde JC, Zickmann B, *et al.* First report on a human percutaneous transluminal implantation of a self-expanding valve prosthesis for interventional treatment of aortic valve stenosis Catheter Cardiovasc Interv 2005; 66: 465-469.

[5]   Andersen HR, Knudsen LL, Hasenkam JM *et al.* Transluminal implantation of artificial heart valves: description of a new expandable aortic valve andinitial results with implantation by catheter technique in closed chest pigs. Eur Heart J. 1992; 13: 704-708.

[6]   Andersen HR *et al.* Transluminal catheter implanted prosthetic heart valves. Int J Angio. 1998; 7: 102-106

[7]   Cribier A, Eltchaninoff H, Bash A, Borenstein N, *et al.* Trans-catheter implantation of balloon-expandable prosthetic heart valves: early results in an animal model. Circulation. 2001; 104(suppl II): I-552.

[8]   Cribier A, Eltcahninoff H, Tron C, *et al.* Early experience with percutaneous transcatheter implantation of the heart valve prosthesis for the treatment of end-stage inoperable patients with calcific aortic stenosis. J Am Coll Cardiol 2004; 43: 698-703.

[9]   Bonow RO, Carabello BA, Kanu C *et al.*ACC/AHA 2006 guideline for management of patient s with valvular hear disease. Circulation 2006; 114 : e84-e231.

[10] Webb JG, Pasupati S, Humphries K. Thompson C, *et al.* Percutaneous Transarterial aortic valve replacement in selected high risk patients with aortic stenosis Circulation, 2007; 116(7): 755-63.

[11] Cribier A, Eltchninoff H, Tron C, Bauer F, *et al.* Percutaneous implantation of aortic valve prosthesis in patients with calcific aortic stenosis: Technical advances, clinical results and future strategies. Journal of Interventional Cardiology. 2006; 19 (SUPPL.5): S87-S96.

[12] Lichtenstein SV, Cheung A, Ye J, *et al.* Transapical transcatheter aortic valve implantation in humans: initial clinical experience Circulation 2006; 114: : 591-596

[13] Grube E, Schuler G, Buellesfeld L, *et al.* Percutaneous aortic valve replacement for severe aortic stenosis in high risk patients using the second- and current third-generation and self expanding corevalve prosthesis: device success and 30 day clinical outcome. J AM Coll Cardiol 2007; 50: 69-76.

[14] Cribier A, Eltcahninoff H, Tron C, *et al.* Treatment of calcific aortic stenosis with the percutaneous heart valve: mid-term follow-up form the intial feasibility studies: the French experience. J Am Coll Cardiol 2006; 47: 1214-1223.

[15] Webb JG, Pasupati S, Humphries K. Thompson C, Altwegg L, Moss R, *et al.* Percutaneous Transarterial aortic valve replacement in selected high risk patients with aortic stenosis Circulation, 2007; 116(7): 755-63.

[16] Svensson LG, Dewey T, Kapadia S, *et al.* United States feasibility study of transcatheter insertion of a stented aortic valve by left ventricular apex. Ann Thorac Surg 2008; 86: 46-54.

[17] Walter T, Simon P, Dewey T *et al.* Transapical minimal invasive aortic valve implantation. Multicentre experience. Circulation 2007 ; 116 : 1-240-5.

[18] Walther T, Falk V, Borger MA, Dewey T, *et al.* Minimally invasive transapical beating heart aortic valve implantation - proof of concept. Eur J Cardiothorac Surg. 2007 ; 31(1) : 9-15.

[19] National Institute for Health and Clinical Excellence. Transcatheter aortic valve implantation for aortic stenosis: guidance. NICE June 2008, IPG 266.

[20] Klein A A, Webb S.T, Tsui S, *et al.* Transcatheter aortic valve insertion: anaesthetic implications of emerging new technology. British Journal of Anaesthesia 2009; 103(6): 792-9.

[21] Walter T, Simon P, Dewey T *et al.* Transapical minimal invasive aortic valve implantation. Multicentre experience. Circulation 2007 ; 116 : 1-240-5.

[22] Otto CM, Mickel MC, Kennedy JW, *et al.* Three tear outcome after balloon aortic valvulopalsty.Insights into prognosis of valavular aortic stenosis. Circulation 1994; 89: 642-650.

[23] Safian RD, Berman AD, Diver DJ *et al*, Balloonaortic valvuloplasty in 170 consecutive patients. N Engl J Med 1988; 319: 125-130.

[24] Percunatneous balloon aortic valvulopalsty. Acute and 30-day follow-up results in 674 patients from NHLBI balloon valvuloplasty Registry. Circulation 1991; 84.

[25] Agarwal A, Kini AS, Attanti S, *et al.* Results of repeat balloon valvuloplasty for treatment of aortic stenosis in patients aged 50-104 years. Am J Cardiol 2005; 95: 43-47.

[26] Lieberman EB, Bashore TM, Hermiller JB, *et al.* Balloon aortic valvuloplasty in adults: failure of procedure to improve long-term survival. J AM Coll Cardiol 1995; 26: 1522-1528.

[27] Eltchaninoff H, Tron C, Bauer F, Brunet D, Baala B, Drogoul L, *et al.* Aortic bioprosthesis implanted percutaneously: three year follow-up. Arch Mal Coeur Vaiss 2007; 100(11): 901, 4-8.

[28] Cribier A, Eltchninoff H, Tron C, Bauer F, *et al.* Percutaneous implantation of aortic valve prosthesis in patients with calcific aortic stenosis: Technical advances, clinical results and future strategies. Journal of Interventional Cardiology. 2006; 19 (SUPPL.5): S87-S96.

[29] Ye J, Cheung A, Lichtenstein SV, Nietlispach F, *et al.* Transapical transcatheter aortic valve implantation: follow-up to 3 years. J Thorac Cardiovasc Surg 2010; 139: 1107-13.

[30] Descoutures F, Himbert D, Lepage L, *et al.* Contemporary surgical or percutaneous management of severe aortic stenosis in the elderly. Eur Heart J. 2008; 29(11): 1410-7.

[31] Grube E, Laborde JC, Gerckens U, *et al.* Percutaneous implantation of the CoreValve self-expanding valve prosthesis in high-risk patients with aortic valve disease: the Siegburg first-in-man study. Circulation 2006; 114: 1616 -24.

[32] Webb JG, Altwegg L, Boone RH, *et al.* Transcatheter aortic valve implantation. Impact on clinical and valve related problems. Circulation 2009; 119: 3009-16.

[33] Tamburino C, Capodanno D, Mul EM, *et al.* Procedural success and 30-day clinical outcomes after percutaneous aortic valve replacement using current third-generation selfexpanding CoreValve prosthesis. J Invasive Cardiol 2009; 21: 93-98

[34] Rodés-Cabau J, Webb JG, Cheung A, *et al.* Transcatheter Aortic Valve Implantation for the Treatment of Severe Symptomatic Aortic Stenosis in Patients at Very High or Prohibitive Surgical Risk Acute and Late Outcomes of the Multicenter Canadian Experience. JACC 2010; 55: 1080-90.

[35] Thomas M, Schymik G, Walther T *et al* on behalf of the Source investigators. Euro PCR 2009 Barcelona.

[36] Tamburino C, Capodanno D, Mulè M, Scarabelli M, Cammalleri V, Barbanti M, Calafiore A, Ussia G. Procedural success and 30-day clinical outcomes after percutaneous aortic valve replacement using current third-generation self-expanding CoreValve prosthesis. J Invasive Cardiol. 2009; 21(3): 99-100.

[37] Buellesfeld L, Wenaweser P, Gerckens U, *et al.* Transcatheter aortic valve implantation: predictors of procedural success—the Siegburg-Bern experience. Eur Heart J; 2010: 31,984-991.

[38] Laborde JC *et al.* Transcatheter aortic valve implantation with the CoreValve ReValving Device. Paper presented at: Transcatheter Cardiovascular Therapeutics; October 12, 2008; Washington, DC.

[39] Schuler G *et al* 'Updates from the Post-CE Approval Multicenter 18 French Expanded Evaluation Registry Using Transarterial Medtronic CoreValve TAVI September 21, 2009 San Francisco.

[40] Walther T, Falk V, Borger MA, Dewey T,*et al.* Minimally invasive transapical beating heart aortic valve implantation - proof of concept. Eur J Cardiothorac Surg. 2007 ; 31(1) : 9-15.

[41] Walther T, Simon P, Dewey T, *et al.* Transapical minimally invasive aortic valve implantation : multicentre experience. Circulation 2007 ; 116(11 Suppl) : 1240-5.

[42] Walther T, Falk V, Kempfert J, Borger MA, *et al.* Transapical minimally invasive aortic valve implantation ; the initial 50 patients. Eur J Cardiothoracic Surg. 2008 ; 33(6) : 983-8.

[43] Walter T, Schuler G, Borger MA, Kempfert J, Seeburger J *et al.* Transapical aortic valve implantation in 100 consecutive patients: comparison to propensity-matched conventional aortic valve replacement. Eur Heart J 2010; 31(11): 1398-403.

[44] Ye J, Cheung A, Lichtenstein SV, Nietlispach F, *et al* Transapical transcatheter aortic valve implantation: follow-up to 3 years. J Thorac Cardiovasc Surg 2010; 139: 1107-13.

[45] Wendler O, Walther T, Nataf P, *et al.* Trans-apical aortic valve implantation: univariate and multivariate analyses of the early results from the SOURCE registry. Eur J Cardiothorac J 2010 ; 38(2) : 119-27.

CHAPTER 4

Valvuloplasty

Patrick A Calvert[1],*, Daniel R Obaid[2],* and Liam M McCormick[3],*

[1]Papworth Hospital, Cambridge, UK; [2]Papworth Hospital, Cambridge, UK; and [3]Papworth Hospital, Cambridge, UK

Abstract: Balloon valvuloplasty is a percutaneous technique that has transformed the lives of thousands of patients disabled by valvular stenosis. However, it is not a panacea for all stenoses and the key to success is in patient selection. Balloon valvuloplasty works best in valves with predominately commissural fusion and little in the way of leaflet thickening or calcification. Young patients with congenital bicuspid aortic or congenital pulmonary valvular stenosis, or any valve with early rheumatic stenosis often have mobile leaflets with commissural fusion. These patients enjoy excellent results from valvuloplasty with extended periods of freedom from re-intervention including surgery [1-5]. Once the valve becomes heavily thickened and calcified, regardless of the original aetiology, not only are the benefits of valvuloplasty reduced, but the risks are also higher. This chapter aims to explain the details behind valvuloplasty of the aortic, mitral and pulmonary valves.

AORTIC STENOSIS

Congenital – Bicuspid Aortic Valve Stenosis

Left ventricular outflow tract obstruction may be sub-valvular, valvular or supra-valvular and may occur diffusely, at single or multiple sites [6]. Frequently, aortic stenosis is part of a more complex congenital disorder. A post-mortem study of 1102 hearts revealed 95 bicuspid aortic valves [7]. 28 occurred in isolation and 67 in association with other cardiac anomalies. 50-80% of patients with coarctation of the aorta and 20.5% of ventricular septal defects also had a bicuspid aortic valve [7,8]. Other associations include patent ductus arteriosus, coronary anatomical variants, Turner's syndrome and Marfan's syndrome [9-13]. This chapter will only deal with isolated valvular causes of aortic stenosis of which the congenital bicuspid aortic valve is the commonest.

The bicuspid aortic valve is one of the commonest congenital cardiac defects with an estimated incidence of 1-2% compared to 0.8% for other congenital cardiac anomalies combined. Only 2% of those with a bicuspid aortic valve will have significant stenosis or regurgitation by adolescence [5]. However, the bicuspid aortic valve undergoes an accelerated degeneration compared to its tricuspid counterpart [14]. Just 20% will maintain normal valve function throughout their live and 30% will suffer serious morbidity including stenosis, regurgitation, infective endocarditis, aortic aneurysm and aortic dissection [14,15].

Aortic stenosis is the commonest complication of a bicuspid aortic valve (6). Stenosis occurs in two-thirds of patients with a bicuspid aortic valve by the fifth decade and makes up greater than 50% of patients with severe aortic stenosis [16-18].

Anatomy

A congenitally bicuspid aortic valve usually consists of two unequal cusps. This usually results in an asymmetric closure line which is clearly visible on echo (depending on the orientation of the closure line). A fibrous band is generally seen in the middle of the larger cusp which marks the point of congenital fusion (Fig. **1a**). This raphe may have a central indentation which can give the false impression of a trileaflet aortic valve [14]. The closure line is usually latero-lateral (Fig. **1a**) rather than antero-posterior (Fig. **1b**) [14]. Greater cusp asymmetry and an antero-posterior closure line are associated with more rapidly progressive stenosis [19]. Classically, the leaflets are said to "dome" in systole (Fig. **1c** and **d**), however, this only occurs if they are mobile and will not occur if cusps are thickened or calcified [1]. In the first three decades of life, the leaflets generally remain thin and mobile with little valve thickening, degeneration or calcification. The stenosis at this stage is predominately related to commissural fusion and therefore balloon valvuloplasty yields excellent results with extended freedom from intervention [20].

*Address correspondence to Patrick A Calvert:** Papworth Hospital, Cambridge, UK; E-mail: Patrick.Calvert@papworth.nhs.uk; E-mail: Daniel.Obaid@papworth.nhs.uk E-mail: Liam.McCormick@papworth.nhs.uk

However, as thickening, degeneration and calcification progress, the stenosed bicuspid aortic valve starts to resemble the senile calcific stenosis of the tricuspid aortic valve and can be difficult to differentiate anatomically. This is discussed further below.

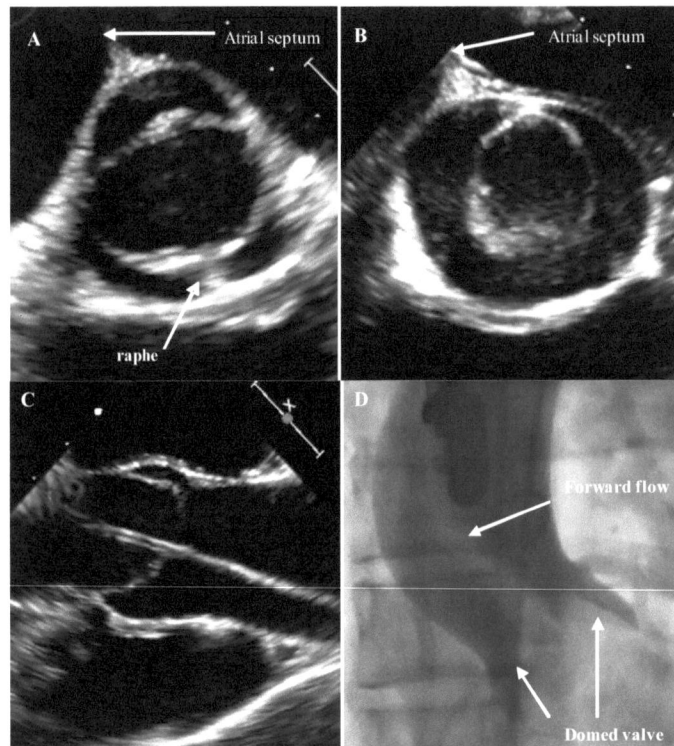

Figure 1: A) Transoesophageal short axis image (60 degrees plane) of a congenital bicuspid aortic valve with a latero-lateral closure line. The raphe in the larger (anterior) cusp is marked. B) Transoesophageal short axis image (40 degrees plane) of a congenital bicuspid aortic valve with antero-posterior closure line. C) Transoesophageal long axis image (102 degrees plane) of a congenital bicuspid aortic valve showing doming of the leaflets. A catheter is seen crossing the valve. D) Aortogram of a congenital bicuspid aortic valve showing doming of the valve and the central forward flow of blood diluting the contrast in the aorta.

Embryology

The semi-lunar valves, the proximal aorta and the pulmonary trunk are all derived from the truncus arteriosus [21,22]. This is formed from the distal third of the bulbus cordis which may form as early as 28 days post-conception and is derived from neural crest cells [23-26]. During the 5th week post-conception, the truncus arteriosus septates to give aortic and pulmonary channels. When partition is almost complete, three tubercles appear in each channel at the proximal end of the truncus arteriosus. Between the 16mm and 40mm embryo stage these tubercles form into the aortic and pulmonary valves [2].

Malformation of the three aortic valve cusps may occur resulting, most commonly, in fusion of two of the cusps. Less common malformations include imperforate aorta, unicuspid and quadracuspid valves [27]. A bicuspid aortic valve results in assymetrical cusps.

Pathophysiology

Malformations of the aortic valve may be thought of as a phenotypic continuum with the thickened unicuspid valve at one end and the rare quadricuspid valve at the other [20]. Several theories attempt to explain the aetiology of aortic valve malformations but none, as yet, predominate. Proponents of an environment cause suggest that differential streaming of blood in the aortic channel of the truncus arteriosus during valvulogenesis results in the asymmetrical cusp formation. However, this explanation remains only a theory.

There is perhaps more substantial evidence supporting a genetic origin. Although bicuspid aortic valves are usually sporadic, family clusters do occur [6-21]. In such cases the inheritance is autosomal dominant with incomplete penetrance [28,29]. The link with Turner's Syndrome (45XO) [30] and the male pre-dominance (male : female ratio 3:1) [31,32] point towards an X-linked inheritance. However, other studies refute the link with the X-chromosome, but do support linkage with chromosomal regions 18q, 5q and 13q [33]. Mutations in the NOTCH-1 gene (chromosome 9q) may not only be responsible for bicuspid aortic valves but also for the accelerated calcium deposits seem in them [34,35].

Another candidate gene is the ubiquitin fusion degradation 1-like (UFD1L) gene which is highly expression in the left ventricular outflow tract during embryogenesis [36]. The locus for UFD1L is on 22q and mutations involving this region results in Di George's syndrome which is associated with bulbus cordis problems including bicuspid aortic valve (amongst other things) [37].

Mutations in the ACTA2 gene (locus 10q) which encodes for vascular smooth muscle cell (VSMCs) alpha-actin is associated with inherited aortic aneurysms and bicuspid aortic valves [38]. Nitric oxide, secreted by VSMCs is important in vascular and valvular embryogenesis and is found in lower levels in the ascending aorta of patients with bicuspid than tricuspid aortic valves [39]. Furthermore, genetically manipulated mice who lack the gene to produce endothelium-derived nitric oxide synthase show an increased in bicuspid aortic valves (5/12 knock-out mice vs. 0/26 controls) [40].

These are just a few of the genes potentially implicated in bicuspid aortic valve and its accelerated degeneration. The myriad of candidate genes suggests that, so far, the true answer eludes us. The actual aetiology may involve a complex interaction of several genes and possibly also environmental factors.

Bicuspid aortic valve stenosis is progressive in the majority of patients. The rate of deterioration is related to the valve anatomy. Severe cusps inequality and unicuspid anatomy leads to rapidly progressive stenosis at an early age [16,17]. This early progression is not only due to the small initial valve orifice but also due to the thickened inflexible cusps and high valve shear stress during systole [41-43]. Even in the normally functioning bicuspid aortic valve, similar forces are at work. Abnormal folding and creasing of the valve, extended areas of valve contact and turbulence occur throughout the cardiac cycle [44].These stress forces lead to valve damage, scarring and eventually restricted motion, calcification and stenosis or regurgitation.

The histopathological findings in a biscuspid aortic valve depend on the initial anatomy and the age of the patient. Those in the first three decades of life may have quite significant valvular stenosis with preservation of good valve architecture and minimal valve thickening or calcification. These patients, in whom the stenosis is largely due to commissural fusion, respond very well to balloon valvuloplasty. However, with time, inflammation, fibrosis, calcification and bone formation occur [16,17,20, 45-49]. By the fifth and sixth decades the stenotic bicuspid aortic valve will have undergone changes very similar to the senile calcific tricuspid aortic valve, albeit one or two decades earlier. Histological changes similar to atherosclerosis have been seen in both biscupid and tricuspid aortic valve stenosis and dyslipidaemia appears to be associated with accelerated stenosis in bicuspid aortic valves [50,51].

Bicuspid Aortic Valve and Aortic Regurgitation

Aortic regurgitation in a bicuspid aortic valve may be due to cusp prolapse or aortic root dilatation. Bicuspid aortic valve is associated with cystic medial necrosis of the aorta, aortic root dilatation and aortic dissection. Studies have demonstrated a variety of collagen abnormalities in the valve and proximal aorta of patients with a bicuspid aortic valve including abnormalities in fibrillin-1, the protein responsible for Marfan's syndrome. However, many of these changes, including cystic medical necrosis, are non-specific. Furthermore, the FBN-1 gene mutation responsible for the fibrillin-1 abnormality in Marfan's syndrome in not found in patients with a bicuspid aortic valve [52].

It is assumed by some that the aortic root dilatations seen in BAV are linked to collagen abnormalities as, in some patients, the associated flow disturbances (stenosis or regurgitation) are too mild to be the sole cause [53]. However mild haemodynamic disturbances have been shown to cause vessel dilatation *in vivo* and in experimental models [54-56]. Although there are small groups with inherited bicuspid aortic valves, the majority are sporadic. The relationship between bicuspid aortic valves, collagen disorders and proximal aortic dilatation remains unclear and is outside the remit of this chapter.

Management

The recommended treatment for severe congenital bicuspid aortic valve stenosis depends on the patient's symptoms, age and the valve anatomy. Young patients (first three decades) with mobile leaflets and commissural fusion without calcification respond well to balloon valvuloplasty [5]. A large registry collected procedural data on 606 patients who underwent aortic valvuloplasty at 23 sites (median age 6.8 year, range 1 month to 18 years). There was a mean reduction in trans-valvular catheter gradient of 60% [57]. The procedural mortality rate was 1.9%. However, this registry included the early learning curve of this procedure as well as a wide variety of valve morphologies.

Medium-term results of a single centre study of 148 patients who underwent valvuloplasty (12 month to 20 years) showed a procedural mortality rate of 0.7% and an 8-year survival of 95% [2]. At 8 years, 70% of patients were free from operation and 50% were free from re-intervention which is similar to results reported from surgical valvuloplasty [5]. In this cohort, 13% of patients had significant regurgitation (grade ≥3/4) post-valvuloplasty compared to 3% pre-procedure. Significant regurgitation (grade ≥3/4) only occurred in 8% of those with trivial or no regurgitation at baseline compared to 33% of those with grade 2/4 regurgitation at baseline.

Any delay in surgery is valuable given the problems inherent with long-term anticoagulation and multiple re-operations. Valvuloplasty also permits children to grow to adult size thus preventing the functional stenosis that arises with prosthesis to body size mismatch. The 2008 American College of Cardiology / American Heart Association guidelines for the management of patients with valvular heart disease make the following class 1 recommendation (evidence level C):

"Aortic balloon valvotomy is indicated in the adolescent or young adult patient with AS [aortic stenosis] who has symptoms of angina, syncope, or dyspnea on exertion and a catheterization peak LV–to–peak aortic gradient greater than or equal to 50 mm Hg without a heavily calcified valve" [5].

Valvulplasty is also a class 1 recommendation (evidence level C) for similar patients with no symptoms but with a gradient greater than 60mmHg [5].

It is worth noting that catheter and echocardiography gradients are usually lower under sedation / general anaesthesia [5].

In patients who are unsuitable for valvuloplasty, then valve repair or replacement is the only effective treatment. Degeneration of homografts in the young is often accelerated and therefore mechanical valves are preferred [5]. The Ross operation, where the patient's own pulmonary valve is transplanted to the aortic position and the pulmonary valve is replaced, has certain theoretical advantages [58, 59]. In particular it permits valve growth in patients who are unsuitable for valvuloplasty. However, it is reported to be a technically challenging operation and there are some concerns regarding autograft dilatation as the pulmonary trunk is derived from the same embryological tissue as the proximal aorta (truncus arteriosus) and may have the same collagen deficiencies [60].

Acquired Senile Calcific Aortic Stenosis

The most common cause of aortic stenosis in the adult population is calcification of the tricuspid (or bicuspid) aortic valve [17, 6-63]. The healthcare burden of severe symptomatic aortic valve stenosis is significant. Best estimates suggest that 1.5% of the elderly population (75-86y) have severe symptomatic aortic stenosis [64]. Only 25% of patients in this age group survive three years after diagnosis compared to 77% of matched controls (65).

Anatomy

Calcific aortic stenosis can be thought of as a continuum with valve thickening and no outflow obstruction (termed aortic sclerosis) at one end and severely thickened, calcified and restricted leaflets at the other (Fig. **2e** and **2f**). The cusps undergo a process of inflammation and lipid accumulation similar to that seen in atherosclerosis [66,67]. At this point the valve may appear thickening without any outflow obstruction. As the process continues the leaflets become restricted and calcification begins, starting at the base of the cusps and progresses to invade the whole leaflet [5]. Eventually the valve is consumed by heavy calcification. The commissures fuse from the base toward the central orifice often creating a "functionally bicuspid" valve.

Pathophysiology

Calcific aortic stenosis used to be termed "degenerative" aortic stenosis with the presumption that calcium was laid down passively after years of "wear and tear". However, there is considerable histopathological evidence that the process involves active inflammation, lipid deposition and calcification in a process similar to atherosclerosis [49].

It is hypothesised that the initial factor in calcific aortic stenosis is endothelial damage due to increased mechanical stresses across the valve[49]. This may explain why bicuspid and rheumatic aortic valves suffer premature calcific aortic stenosis. In each leaflet, extra-cellular lipid accumulation and lipoproteins are seen [66,67] Oxidated low density lipoproteins are taken up by macrophages which become foam cells [68]. In the early process, inflammatory cells predominate, in particular T-cells, macrophages and monocytes [66, 69-71]. Activated T-cells within the subendothelium release pro- inflammatory cytokines such as interleukin-1ß which promotes local synthesis of matrix metalloproteins which facilitate extra-cellular matrix formation and calcification [72]. The chain of events seen in calcific aortic stenosis are directly analagous to atherosclerosis and are seen as early as aortic sclerosis [49].

HMG-CoA reductase inhibitors (statins) are known to be anti-inflammatory as well as lowering serum lipids levels [73]. Statins are not only able to reduced atherosclerotic plaque burden [74, 75] but they can also change plaque composition, potential stabilizing the process [76]. Given the similarities between the two disease processes it is logical to assume that statins may also slow the progression of aortic stenosis. Retrospective studies

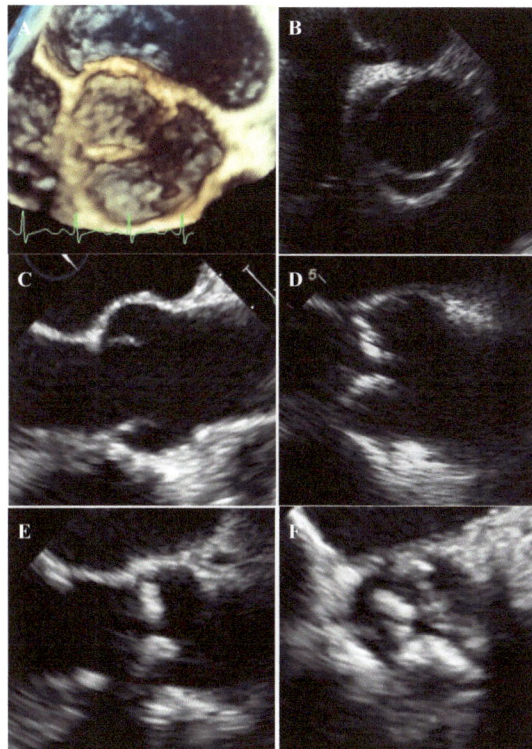

Figure 2: A) Three dimension transoesophageal short axis image of a normal aortic valve in diastolic. B) Transoesophageal short axis image of a normal aortic valve in systole. C) Transoesophageal long axis image of a normal aortic valve in systole. D) Transoesophageal long axis image of a severe stenosed aortic valve in systole. This valve is only mildly thickened with no real calcification but opening is severely restricted secondary to field radiotherapy. E) Transoesophageal long axis image of a severely stenosed and thickened aortic valve in systole with moderately calcification. F) Transoesophageal short axis image of a severely stenosed, thickened and calificied aortic valve in systole

have suggested a potential role for statins in aortic stenosis [77,78]. However, a randomized contolled trial of simvastatin and ezetimibe versus placebo in mild to moderate aortic stenosis showed a reduction in ischaemic cardiac events but no reduction in patients' requirement for aortic valve replacement [79]. It is possible that the follow up (median 52 month) was too short to demonstrate a benefit or that the disease process is only modifiable in the early stages of aortic sclerosis. An equally plausible theory, however, is that the observed shared processes between aortic stenosis and atherosclerosis are part of a repair mechanism responding to an, as yet unidentified, injurious stimulus.

Management

The only efficacious treatment for severe symptomatic, calcific aortic stenosis is valve replacement. Once the patient develops symptoms (exertional dyspnoea, angina or syncope) the average survival is two to three years with a high risk of sudden death [80-83]. No prospective studies have been performed randomising patients to valve replacement or placebo, as this would be unethical. However, the uncontrolled data we have suggests that valve replacement returns the patient survival curve back to that of matched controls with good survival rates post surgery, even in the elderly [80, 84].

A large proportion (33-60%) of patients with symptomatic severe aortic stenosis do not undergo surgery, often because of perceived high operative risk [85-88]. Transcatheter aortic valve implantation (TAVI) was developed to fill this unmet clinical need and is discussed further in the TAVI chapter [89-95].

Although valvuloplasty plays and an important part in the treatment of congenital aortic stenosis in children and young adults, its role in the management of calcified aortic stenosis is very limited [5]. Valvuloplasty works in this population by fracturing calcium deposits and to a lesser extent stretching the annulus and splitting commissures [96-98]. Haemodynamic improvements are small and valve area rarely exceed $1.0cm^2$ post-procedure. Despite the modest improvement in valve area, the patients typically enjoy a significant but short-lived improvement in symptoms [99-104]. The symptomatic benefit of valvuloplasty in these patients lasts no more than 6-12 months. Although there are no prospective, randomised controlled trials, registry data suggest that survival is no better than medical therapy alone[103,105]. Significant complications rates are approximately 10% and include death, stroke, heart block, acute valvular regurgitation and vascular injury [99, 106-108].

Acquired Rheumatic Aortic Stenosis

Rheumatic fever results in a pan-carditis in 50% of cases [109]. Inflammation and subsequent scarring of the valves and mitral sub-valvular apparatus occurs. Although the mitral valve is most commonly affected, the aortic valve may also be involved. The resultant valve anatomy and therefore dysfunction depends on the degree and duration of scarring. If stenosis is largely due to commissural fusion rather than valve thickening or calcification, then such patients may respond very well to valvuloplasty (both aortic and mitral). However, if the cusps are heavily thickened and calcified or if there is moderate or worse regurgitation, then valvuloplasty is not an option.

Aortic Valvuloplasty - the Procedure

In adults, the procedure can be performed under local anaesthesia (with or without light sedation) in a standard catheter laboratory. As for any procedure, the patient should be properly informed of the expected benefits and potential risks, prior to the procedure and given opportunity to discuss issues with family member. This is particular important for calcific aortic stenosis where the risk benefit analysis may be marginal.

Careful planning in advance reduces the risk of procedural complications. The pre-procedural transthoracic echocardiogram should be studied in advance to determine the aetiology of the stenosis, degree of calcification and regurgitation. All of these factors should be taken into account when attempting to predict the overall risks of the procedure. We would not recommend performing valvuloplasty on a patient who has more than 2/4 regurgitation. Left ventricular impairment contributes to the risk of the proceedure as patients are less likely to tolerate rapid pacing and left ventricular outflow tract occlusion with a balloon. Left ventricular thrombus is an absolute contra-indication to aortic valvuloplasty.

The aortic annulus size should be carefully measured as this will determine the size of the balloon. Analysis of 630 valvuloplasties in children and young adults determined the optimal balloon to annulus ratio = 0.9-1.0 [57].

Undersizing rendered the procedure ineffective whereas oversizing resulted in regurgitation complications. These ratios are validated for non-calcified congenital aortic stenotic valves. The calcified valves pose a greater risk of regurgitation and a more conservative ratio is advised. A number of high pressure balloons are available in the UK, including the Cristal Balloon (Pyramed Ltd, UK) and the Z-Med™ Balloon (NuMED Inc, Hopkinton NY). Both balloons come in various sizes and are actually quite compliant with a broad range of size depending on the pressure generated by the indeflator or syringe. This makes accurate sizing of the balloon difficult. The large volume required to fill the balloon and the rapidity at which inflation must occur, means that a specialized indeflator such as those used in TAVI procedures or a 30ml syringe must be used.

Physiological monitoring is required with two pressure lines, pulse oximetry and electrocardiogram. Transthoracic echocardiography is recommended to assess for gradient reduction, regurgitation and pericardial effusion. An intravenous "long-line" is useful to ease the administration of drugs as they are required.

Access is gained in a femoral vein and a temporary pacing wire is placed at the right ventricular apex. Bilateral femoral artery access gives the best peak to peak trans-aortic monitoring and permits aortograms to be performed to assess for regurgitation. However, if femoral access is difficult on one side, transvalvular pressures can be measure from the side-arm of an over-sized sheath in the femoral artery or upon catheter pull-back across the aortic valve. A 10-14F sheath is required to accommodate the valvuloplasty balloon depending on its size and make.

The stenosed aortic valve is crossed retrogradially. This is most easily done with a standard weight 0.035 inch straight tipped wire in an Amplatzer left one diagnostic catheter (vertical root) or an Amplatzer left two diagnostic catheter (horizontal root eg unfolded aorta). Some operators used a technique of "mapping" the valve as was first described by Alain Cribier.

Once the catheter is in the left ventricle it can be used to measure peak to peak gradients between its tip and that of a pigtail catheter placed in the aortic root *via* the other groin arterial access. The soft tip of an Amplatzer extra-stiff exchange length wire should then be shaped into a large curve. This is then placed in the left ventricle *via* the Amplatzer left one catheter, which is removed leaving the extra-stiff wire in situ across the aortic valve. The valvulplasty balloon is de-air and attached to an indeflator or syringe with the correct amount of dilute (one fifth strength) radio-opaque contrast to generate the required stretch diameter. The balloon is then place in the ascending aorta. Rapid right ventricular pacing (180-210pbm) is then tested to ensure 1:1 capture occurs so that the aortic pressure drops to approximately 40mmHg with minimal systolic rise. Without these conditions, the balloon will be unstable moving distally on systole thus risking damage to the aortic valve and aorta.

Rapid pacing and balloon inflation in the left ventricular outflow tract can precipitate cardiac decompensation, especially in those with poor ventricular function. Therefore, it is recommended that a systolic pressure greater 100mmHg is achieved using inotropes before valvuloplasty is attempted.

Having notified the catheter laboratory staff of your intention to proceed to valvuloplasty, you advance the balloon so that it is centred on the calcification of the valve (this usually results in a small drop in blood pressure) (Fig. **3**). Rapid pacing is commenced and when the blood pressure is low and stable the balloon is fully and rapidly inflated (Fig. **4**) and then deflated before rapid pacing is ceased. Fine movements of the balloon may be required to prevent it from prolapsing off the valve. As soon as the balloon is deflated, remove it away from the valve to aid pressure recovery. The sonographer can assess for new regurgitation as well as reduction in the gradient whilst the blood pressure recovers. If there is no heart block, no increase in regurgitation and the pressure recovers quickly and completely the procedure may be repeated if required. Assessment of regurgitation and trans-valvular gradient should be repeated on catheter measurements.

Assessment of haemodynamic measurements (both catheter and echocardiographically) can be difficult, especially if the patient is sedated. The decision to perform repeated balloon inflations or cease the procedure must be made on a case by case basis. Although significant reductions in gradients may be seen in young adults with non-calcified congenital aortic stenosis, the reduction in the gradient in older calcified valves is often modest.

The temporary pacing wire should remain in situ for approximately 24 hours and arterial haemostasis should ideally be achieved by any of a variety of commercially available closure devices.

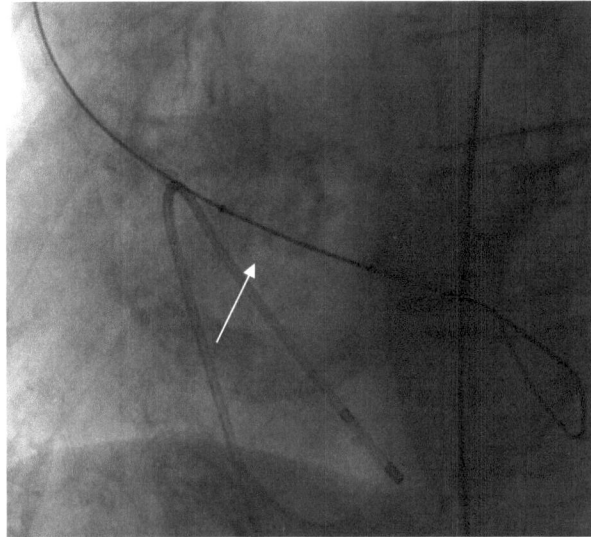

Figure 3: Left anterior oblique view. The valvuloplasty balloon has been centre on the aortic valve calcification (arrow), by passing it over an Amplatzer extra-stiff exchange length wire. A temporary pacing wire has been placed at the right ventricular apex.

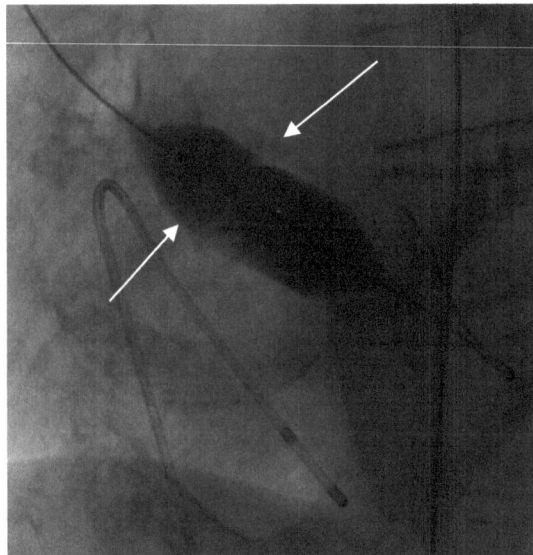

Figure 4: Left anterior oblique view. The same patient and view as for Fig. 3. The valvuloplasty balloon is inflated during rapid right ventricular pacing. The calcified aortic valve can be seen indenting the balloon (arrows).

MITRAL STENOSIS

Mitral stenosis was first described by the French physician Vieussens more than 300 years ago and has traditionally been responsible for significant morbidity and mortality. In developed countries its incidence has decreased in modern times due to a reduction in the prevalence of rheumatic fever, its main causal agent. Despite this, it remains important for the modern cardiologist to retain an understanding of this condition as patients will continue to present following emigration from developing countries where rheumatic fever remains endemic. In addition some patients from developed countries continue to develop mitral stenosis although the pattern of disease is changing. Previously, only surgery could provide any form of relief of the valve obstruction. However, in the last 25 years percutaneous balloon mitral valvuloplasty (PBMV) has proven to be an effective therapy in appropriately selected patients. Its use has expanded and it is currently considered to be the therapy of choice for symptomatic patients with severe mitral stenosis who have appropriate valvular anatomy for the procedure.

Aetiology

Traditionally, virtually all acquired mitral stenosis has been ascribed to rheumatic heart disease. In previous surgical and pathological series, rheumatic involvement has been found in 99% of mitral valves excised for stenosis [110,111]. This remains the case in developing countries where rheumatic fever is endemic. In contrast, in developed countries there has been a steady fall in the prevalence of rheumatic fever over the last century (0.6% of schoolchildren in India compared with 0.05% in developed countries) [112]. This has led to a corresponding fall in the prevalence of mitral stenosis in developed countries. In one European centre, mitral stenosis accounted for 9% of valvular disease in 1985 compared with 43% in 1960 [113]. Despite the reduction in the incidence of rheumatic fever it was still responsible for the majority of cases of mitral stenosis in a recent large multi-centre European registry, accounting for 85% of adult presentations [114]. Mitral stenosis accounted for 10% of all valve cases in this series and it has been suggested that this is unlikely to diminish further given current immigration patterns [115]. Therefore the treatment of mitral stenosis will remain relevant for cardiologists in developed countries.

Other causes of mitral stenosis make up only a small proportion of the total burden. In the "Euro Heart Survery", degenerative mitral valve disease was reported as the cause of 12.5% of the cases of mitral stenosis [114]. The extensive calcification of the mitral annulus that occurs in degenerative mitral valves is more commonly associated with mitral regurgitation [116]. However, it causes significant stenosis in some patients [117]. Given the decline in rheumatic heart disease and the increase in life expectancy, the proportion of mitral stenosis cases attributed to calcific degenerative disease is likely to increased [118].

The remaining causes of mitral stenosis make up less than 3% of all cases [114]. These include congenital causes (often presenting in infancy) such as shortened chordae, parachute mitral valve, double mitral orifice and supra-mitral ring [119]. Often these are seen in association with other congenital abnormalities and median age of death without treatment is 2 months [120]. Systemic conditions such as rheumatoid arthritis and systemic lupus erythematosis can cause mitral stenosis on rare occasions. Mitral stenosis has also been described in carcinoid [121], Fabry's disease [122] and infective endocarditis[123]. Mitral stenosis may be iatrogenic, for example mitral annuloplasty, following previous surgical commisurotomy or methysergide treatment.

Pathology

Rheumatic heart disease is a late sequela of rheumatic fever. The initial infective episode is a pharyngitis caused by group A beta-haemolytic streptococcus. This is followed some weeks later by a systemic inflammatory response. Widespread foci of fibrinoid necrosis occur, although the presence of these areas termed "Aschoff bodies" are found only infrequently in the heart where they are considered pathognomonic of rheumatic carditis. They appear to be more prevalent in cases where the mitral valve is affected [124].

The initial episode results in verruciform deposition of fibrin along the closure lines of the mitral valve. These acute valvular changes usually resolve with little disturbance to cardiac function. However, in susceptible individuals there follows progressive damage to the valve, probably secondary to a chronic inflammatory response [125]. This chronic inflammatory response may be perpetuated by T lymphocyte mimicry between streptococcal M protein and cardiac myosin [126]. This inflammation combined with chronic haemodynamic injury leads to progressive stenosis of the mitral valve which occurs over many years with leaflet thickening, commissural fusion and shortening, thickening and fusion of the chordae tendinae. This causes the mitral valve orifice to take on the classic slit like "fish mouth" appearance characteristic of rheumatic mitral stenosis (Fig. **5**). Other valves may become involved, however the mitral valve, either singly or in combination with another valve is by far the most common site affected by rheumatic heart disease.

Improvements in echocardiographic technology means that degenerative mitral stenosis is diagnosed more frequently than previously [118]. It is pathologically quite distinct from rheumatic mitral valve disease with relative sparring of the leaflet tips and commissures and extensive calcification of the mitral valve annulus [127]. This difference is important when considering suitability for PBMV which will be discussed later. It is unusual for mitral annular calcification to cause haemodynamically significant mitral stenosis, however where there is extensive mitral annular calcification, calcium encroaching on to the valve leaflets and impinging opening causes stenosis in 6-8% of cases [128]. Other possible mechanisms of stenosis with annular calcification are reduction of normal mitral annular dilatation during diastole [129,30] and impaired anterior mitral leaflet mobility[131].

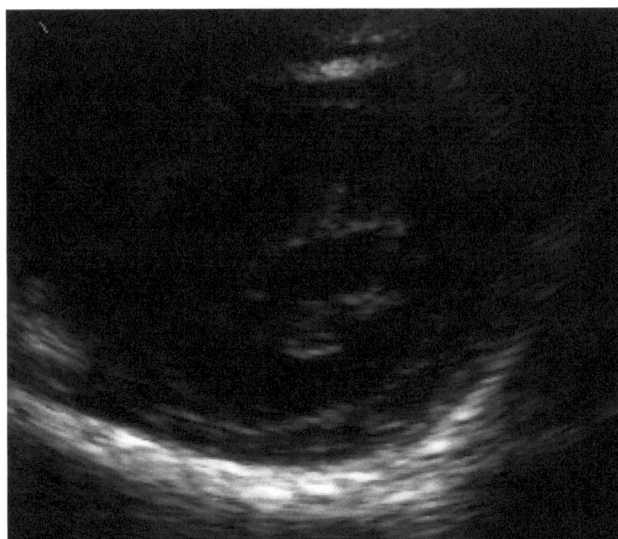

Figure 5: Transthoracic echocardiogram (short axis) of a mitral valve with rheumatic stenosis cut at the leaflet tips in late diastole. Thickening of the leaflet tips and the classic "fish-mouth" mitral orifice are clearly seen.

Natural History

The natural history of rheumatic mitral stenosis has been well characterised from studies performed over 4 decades ago [132,133]There is a latent phase between initial infection and the development of symptoms of mitral stenosis. This latent phase varies in length, however it tends to be shorter in developing countries requiring intervention earlier [134]. The mean age of presentation with rheumatic mitral stenosis in a study of Indian patients was 15.1 years. [112]. This contrasts with a much longer disease progression seen in developed countries [135] and is felt to be due to the effect of repeated episodes of infection in developing countries. In north America and Europe, the mean age of presentation with mitral stenosis in the fifth or sixth decade [136.115].

Patients with degenerative mitral stenosis tend to present at older ages and with less severe stenosis [118]. The development of mitral annular calcification is not only associated with increasing age, it is also associated with significant co-morbidities such as hypertension, aortic stenosis, renal failure, diabetes mellitus and coronary artery disease [137, 138, 139]. This makes these patients higher risk for surgical treatment. In addition, the morphology of the stenosed mitral valve often prohibits PBMV.

Pathophysiology

The characteristic pathophysiological feature of mitral stenosis is an obstruction to left ventricular in-flow at the level of the mitral valve as a result of a structural abnormality of the mitral valve plus minus apparatus. The primary abnormality is of impairment of diastolic filling of the left ventricle. However, as the disease progresses there are secondary consequences on the left atrium and pulmonary vasculature, caused by the elevated transmitral gradient.

The normal mitral valve area is 4.0 to 5.0 cm^2. Symptoms at rest are not usually apparent until this has narrowed to less then 1.5 cm^2. At this stage the cardiac output is impaired at rest [140]. However, symptoms may occur before this stage as cardiac output fails to rise effectively. Symptoms can be precipitated by conditions that cause tachycardia (by reducing diastolic filling time) or that require an increase in cardiac output, for example exercise, infection, pregnancy and atrial fibrillation [141].

In mitral stenosis, a reduction in valve area necessitates development of a transmitral gradient to allow blod to flow from the left atrium to the left ventricle [142]. Chronic elevation of left atrial pressure leads to chamber enlargement and remodeling which predisposes to the development of atrial arrhythmias. Atrial fibrillation greatly increases the risk of systemic thrombo-emboli and reduces cardiac output and exercise capacity. It is present in 40-75% of patients who present with symptomatic mitral stenosis [143,144].

The other consequence of chronically elevated left atrial pressure is an increase in pulmonary artery pressure. Pulmonary hypertension is a common finding in severe mitral stenosis and factors shown to affect the pulmonary vascular bed gradient were transmitral pressure gradient, left ventricular end-diastolic pressure, mitral valve area and a previous history of chronic pulmonary disease [145]. In untreated mitral stenosis, severe pulmonary hypertension is associated with poor prognosis, with a mean survival of less than 3 years [146]. Pulmonary hypertension often improves following surgery or PBMV (147). However, this improvement is often incomplete (148). The presence of pulmonary hypertension pre-PBMV has been identified as an independent predictor of adverse events following treatment [149].

Management

Drug treatment for patients in sinus rhythm with symptomatic mitral stenosis is limited to palliation by slowing heart rate to increase left ventricular filling in diastole and diuretic therapy to reduce pulmonary congestion. Initial attempts at relieving the stenosis by performing surgical valvotomy where described by Cutler in 1923 [150] and an attempt at comissurotomy by Suttar in 1925 (151). Invasive therapies did not become common place until the first closed commissurotomies described by Bailey and Harken in the 1940's [152] [153]. Following the development of cardiopulmonary bypass this was largely replaced by open surgical commissurotomy. The principle behind both techniques was to decrease the amount of stenosis by causing a split between the fused commissures without fracture of the valve leaflets or damage to the sub valvular apparatus which causes significant mitral regurgitation. Percutaneous treatment began in 1982 when Japanese surgeon Kanji Inoue described the first percutaneous balloon mitral valvuloplasty [154]. The principle was to inflate a balloon inserted percutaneously into the mitral valve in order to split the fused commissures and increase leaflet mobility and valve area. Splitting of commissures was later proven to be the results of the balloon inflation and was sometimes accompanied by cracking of calcification [155, 156].

Selection of Patients for Percutaneous Balloon Mitral Valvuloplasty

It is vital to the success of PBMV that only patients with appropriate valve anatomy are selected to undergo the procedure. There are commonly four factors that influence whether a patient with mitral stenosis should be considered for PBMV:

1. The stenosis should be severe enough to warrant intervention (mitral stenosis is considered severe when the valve area < 1.0 cm^2. However other haemodynamic variables including pulmonary artery pressure are also considered.

2. The patient should have symptoms severe enough to warrant intervention.

3. The anatomy of the mitral valve should be suitable for PBMV. The best results are seen in patients with stenosis due to fused commissures, with non-calcified valves, pliable leaflets and minimal involvement of the sub-valvular apparatus.

4. There should be no contraindications to PBMV.

Recent guidelines outlining which patients should be considered for PBMV have been published jointly by the American Heart Association and American College of Cardiology [5].

They consider that PBMV should be performed in:

1. Symptomatic patients (NYHA functional class II, III, or IV), with moderate or severe mitral stenosis and valve morphology favorable for PBMV in the absence of left atrial thrombus or moderate to severe mitral regurgitation. (Class I recommendation level of evidence: A)

2. Asymptomatic patients with moderate or severe mitral stenosis and valve morphology that is favorable for percutaneous mitral balloon valvotomy who have pulmonary hypertension (pulmonary artery systolic pressure greater than 50 mm Hg at rest or greater than 60 mmHg with exercise) in the absence of left atrial thrombus or moderate to severe mitral regurgitation [5]. (Class I recommendation level of evidence: C)

It is reasonable to perform PBMV in:

1. Patients with moderate or severe mitral stenosis who have a non-pliable calcified valve, who are in NYHA functional class III–IV, and are either not candidates for surgery

    or are at high surgical risk [5]. Class IIa recommendation level of evidence: C)

PBMV may be considered in:

1. Asymptomatic patients with moderate or severe mitral stenosis and valve morphology favorable for percutaneous mitral balloon valvotomy who have new onset of atrial fibrillation in the absence of left atrial thrombus or moderate to severe mitral regurgitation. (Class IIb recommendation level of evidence: C)

2. Symptomatic patients (NYHA functional class II, III, or IV) with mitral valve area greater than 1.5 cm^2 if there is evidence of haemodynamically significant MS based on pulmonary artery systolic pressure greater than 60 mm Hg, pulmonary artery wedge pressure of 25 mm Hg or more, or mean mitral valve gradient greater than 15 mm Hg during exercise. (Class IIb recommendation level of evidence: C)

3. As an alternative to surgery for patients with moderate or severe mitral stenosis who have a non-pliable calcified valve and are in NYHA functional class III-IV.[5]. (Class IIb recommendation level of evidence: C)

PBMV should not be performed in:

1   Patients with mild mitral stenosis. (Class III recommendation level of evidence: C)

2   Patients with moderate to severe mitral regurgitation or left atrial thrombus [5]. (Class III recommendation level of evidence: C)

Echocardiographic Evaluation

Transthoracic echocardiography is considered mandatory for the diagnosis of mitral stenosis and also to assess haemodynamic severity (mean gradient, mitral valve area and pulmonary artery pressure). It also assists in the assessment of the morphology of the mitral valve, and to look for other concommitant valvular lesions. If PBMV is considered then transoesophageal echocardiography should be performed to further evaluate the morphology of the mitral valve, accurately quantify any mitral regurgitation and look for the presence of left atrial thrombus. The subvalvular apparatus is often better seen on transoesophgeal echocardiography [5].

The most widely used echocardiographic approach to evaluate the mitral valve morphology is the mitral echocardiographic scoring system devised by Wilkins *et al.* [157] (Table **1**). This system involves allocating a score between 1 and 4 for four different aspects of the valve morphology. The lowest possible score is 4 and the highest is 16. A score of <8 is considered to give the best results with PBMC and a score >12 potentially predicts poorer results and these patient should only be considered for PBMC if they are unsuitable for surgery. The Wilkens score was only based upon 22 patients undergoing PBMV and therefore may have limited validity. A further limitation of using this scoring system is that it does not take into account the anatomy of the commissures, a significant feature given that splitting of the commissures is vital to the success of the procedure. Fatkin *et al.* showed that commissural splitting could be predicted from the pre-procedure echocardiogram and was a better predictor of a good outcome than the mitral echocardiographic score [158]. Sutaria *et al.* showed that commissural calcification was associated with only a 50% likelihood of achieving a post procedure valve area > 1.5cm^2 [159].

Cardiac Catheterisation

Cardiac catheterisation is not routinely recommended unless there is suboptimal echocardiograhic data to assess the severity and haemodynamic status of the mitral stenosis. Catheterisation is also useful if the echo derived data is in conflict with the physical findings or severity of symptoms. Catheterisation should be performed in older patients or in those with risk factors for coronary artery disease as the co-existence of coronary disease requiring surgical revascularisation would be an indication for surgical treatment or mitral stenosis [5].

Table 1: The Wilkens mitral echocardiopgrahic score. Adapted from Wilkens *et al.* (157)

Score	Mobility
1	Leaflet tips only restricted
2	Normal mobility of mid and basal leaflets
3	Valve leaflets move forward in diastole mainly from the base
4	Minimal or no forward movement of leaflets in diastole
	Valvular thickening
1	Near normal thickness (4-5mm)
2	Mid-leaflets normal, margins are considerable thickened (5-8mm)
3	Thickening extends throughout the entire leaflet (5-8mm)
4	Extensive thickening of all leaflet tissue (>8-10mm)
	Subvalvular thickening
1	Minimal thickening
2	Thickening of chordae extending up to one third of chordal length
3	Thickening extending to the distal third of the chords
4	Widespread thickening and shortening involving all chordal structures extending to the papillary muscles
	Calcification
1	Single area of increased echogenicity
2	Scattered areas of echo brightness confined to leaflet margins
3	Echo brightness extending to the mid-portion of the leaflets
4	Extensive echo brightness throughout much of the leaflet tissue

Contraindications to Percutaneous Balloon Mitral Valvuloplasty

There are four main contraindications to PBMV:

Thrombus

Left atrial thrombus is considered a contraindication to PBMV due to the danger of embolisation following instrumentation. Transoesophageal echo is the modality of choice to detect left atrial thrombus [160]. Most operators believe left atrial thrombus is an absolute contraindication to PBMV. If thrombus is still present despite a period of anti-coagulation at higher than normal INR ranges, surgical intervention is generally indication [161]. Although there are reports of PBMV being performed safely in cases of left atrial thrombus [162], it remains a contraindication in the most recently published guidelines [5].

Mitral Regurgitation

Mitral regurgitation greater then 2/4 is also considered a contraindication to PBMV under current guidelines [5]. Patient with pre-existing moderate mitral regurgitation will achieve similar increases in mitral valve area as those with lesser regurgitation, but this is at the expense of an increased risk of severe regurgitation [163]. Long-term follow up (mean 33 months) reveals that pre-existing mitral regurgitation was shown to be an independent predictor of adverse events [164].

Severe Calcification

Given that successful PBMV relies upon the splitting of fused commissures it is unsurprising that calcification of the commissures can impact on potential success. In patients with symmetrical calcification of the commissures, there may be no splitting and hence no response at all to PBMV [158]. Severe calcification of the mitral valve leaflets has also been shown to predict the occurrence of severe mitral regurgitation which is due to leaflet tearing [165].

Pathological examination of mitral valve following failed PBMV demonstrated that asymmetrical calcification was associated with leaflet tearing [166]. Although significant mitral valve calcification dictates that the valve morphology is unfavourable for PBMV, this is a relative rather than absolute contra-indication. As will be discussed later, there is a population of elderly patients that are unsuitable for surgery that may benefit from palliation of symptoms using PMBV.

Aortic Stenosis or Coronary Artery Disease Requiring Surgery

Patients requiring open heart surgery for other valvular lesions or for coronary revascularisation should be considered for surgical commissurotomy or mitral valve replacement during the same operation.

The Inoue Technique

The Inoue balloon catheter system was the first to be developed for non-surgical mitral commissurotomy [154] and is now the commonest method of PBMV in most parts of the world [161]. Japanese surgeon Kanji Inoue first developed a double lumen balloon to perform atrial septostomy in children with cyanotic congenital heart disease [167]. He then evaluated its ability to split fused mitral valve commissures under direct vision in an open surgical commissurotomy [168]. The Inoue balloon catheter (IBC) (Toray Medical, Tokyo, Japan) consists of a rubber balloon covered with a nylon mesh on a polyvinyl chloride tube shaft with a coaxial double lumen. The balloon's profile can be reduced by inserting the "balloon stretch tube" into the outer lumen (Fig. 7). The Inoue balloon also has a compliance curve that allows it to dilate over at least a 4mm range of sizes, depending upon the inflating volume.

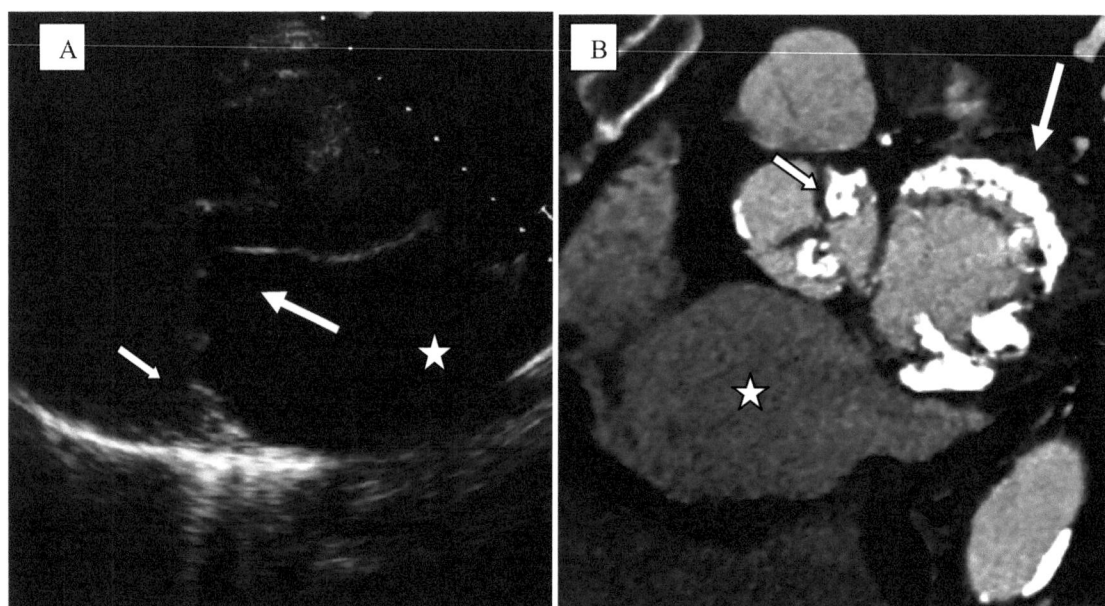

Figure 6: A) Parasternal long axis transthoracic echocardiogram demonstrating rheumatic mitral stenosis with favourable anatomy for PBMV: large arrow – flexible leaflets (as evidenced by doming) with minimal thickening, small arrow – minimal subvalvular thickening. B) Cardiac CT demonstrating degenerative mitral valve disease with unfavourable anatomy for PBMV: large arrow – significant annular calcification extending onto leaflets. Small arrow shows co-existing aortic calcification. Star demonstrates enlarged left atrium (a consequence of mitral stenosis in both images).

Uniquely, the balloon has 3 segments with different compliance so that as it is inflated the distal portion dilates first, followed by the proximal portion and then finally the middle portion. This attribute facilitates fixation of the catheter in the mitral valve orifice. Balloon sizing is the key to procedural success as too small a balloon will result in ineffective dilatation, and too large a balloon risks regurgitation. The balloon is available in a variety of sizes (24mm, 26mm, 28mm and 30mm). Standard practice is to choose balloon size depending on the height of the patient, with allowances made for very diseased valves or patients of advanced age [169]. Some authors maintain that the balloon should be sized using two-dimensional measurements obtained by echocardiography to reduce the risk of over-sizing [161].

The procedure can be performed under local anaesthesia in a standard catheter laboratory. It recommended that moderate sedation is used as parts of the procedure may be uncomfortable. An intravenous "long-line" is useful to ease the administration of drugs as they are required. Physiological monitoring is required with two pressure lines, pulse oximetry and electrocardiogram. Transthoracic echocardiography is recommended to assess for gradient reduction, regurgitation and pericardial effusion.

We will describe the almost universally used anterograde transseptal Inoue technique, although a retrograde arterial approach has been described [170]. Refer to Fig. **7** for details of the IBC nomenclature. Arterial access is gained in a femoral artery with a 6F sheath and an arterial blood oxygen saturation is measured. Coronary anatomy should be delineated if not previously done. A pigtail catheter is placed in the left ventricle where it will remain until the end of the procedure to give continuous direct trans-mitral gradients. A left ventriculogram is performed with right anterior oblique angulation. This helps confirm the degree of baseline regurgitation as well as define the longitudinal axis of the left ventricle down which the Inoue balloon must travel.

Name of set item	Purpose
① Inoue Balloon Catheter (IBC)	Dilation of valve
② Balloon stretching tube	Elongation of balloon
③ Dilator	Dilation of the femoral vein puncture site and the interatrial septum
④ Guidewire	Guiding of catheter and dilator
⑤ Stylet (Spring)	Directing balloon to valve
⑥ Syringe	Inflation of balloon
⑦ Ruler	Measurement of balloon diameter

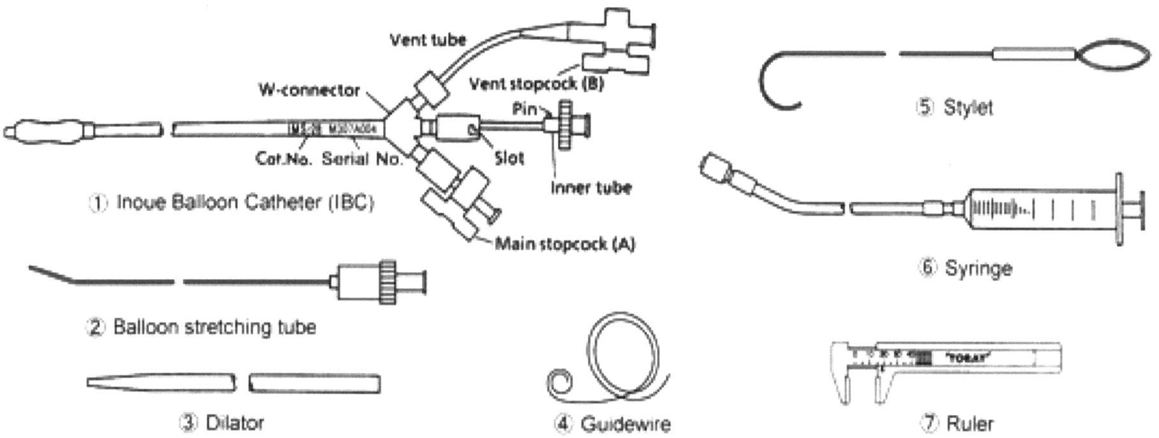

Figure 7: Schematic of the Inoue Balloon Catheter. Reproduced with permission of Toray Medical, Tokyo, Japan.

A 7F sheath is introduced into the right femoral vein with a large skin incision (1cm) and the pulmonary artery pressure is measured and a mixed venous blood oxygen saturation is measured. This route of access is then used to perform the transseptal puncture. The technique described below is used by experienced operators with low complication rates. However, it is recommended that less experienced operators use transoesophageal echocardiography to guide the transseptal puncure. This has the added benefit of more accurately selecting a low atrial septal puncture which makes it easier to introducing the Inoue system into the mitral valve orifice than a high puncture.

The femoral venous sheath is exchanged for any of a variety of commercial available transseptal sheaths (preferably without side-holes as the "curly" Inoue guidewire can get entangled in these). The transseptal sheath is passed over the 0.035 inch standard weight guidewire into the superior vena cava. The guidewire is removed and a Brockenbrough needle is inserted into the lumen of the obturator transseptal sheath until it lies 1cm short of its tip. The needle is then attached to a pressure line. The side-arm of the transseptal sheath and the arrow on the needle should be aligned at an angle of approximately "4 o'clock". With a 20 degree left anterior oblique angulation on fluoroscopy, the transseptal sheath is moved slowly from the superior vena cava into the right atrium, at which point the tip of the sheath will be felt (and seen) to move forward slightly as it falls into the right atrium. After moving the sheath approximately a further 1-2 cm inferiorly, the tip of the needle should move forward again as it falls into the ovale fossa. If there is no ridge at the superior junction between the secundum and primum atria septa then this will not occur (estimated to be the case in approximately 10% of ovale fossae). This second movement suggests that the needle tip is at the superior margin of the ovale fossa. Advancement of the sheath (wide needle back from the tip) may push it through a patent foramen ovale. However, these are usually antero-superior in the ovale fossa and a more antero-inferior position is required to give good access to the mitral orifice. This can be achieved by drawing the sheath approximately 1cm more inferiorly.

Advancing the sheath alone at this point should cause the right atrial pressure trace to damp as it comes into contact with the ovale fossa. If you are satisfied with your position, then advance the needle whilst watching the pressure tracing. With the needle full advanced, it should project approximately 1cm beyond the tip of the transseptal sheath's obturator. Only advance the sheath over the needle if you have a good left atrial pressure trace (higher that the right atrial pressure). If there is any doubt then pull the needle back into the sheath and start again from the superior vena cava.

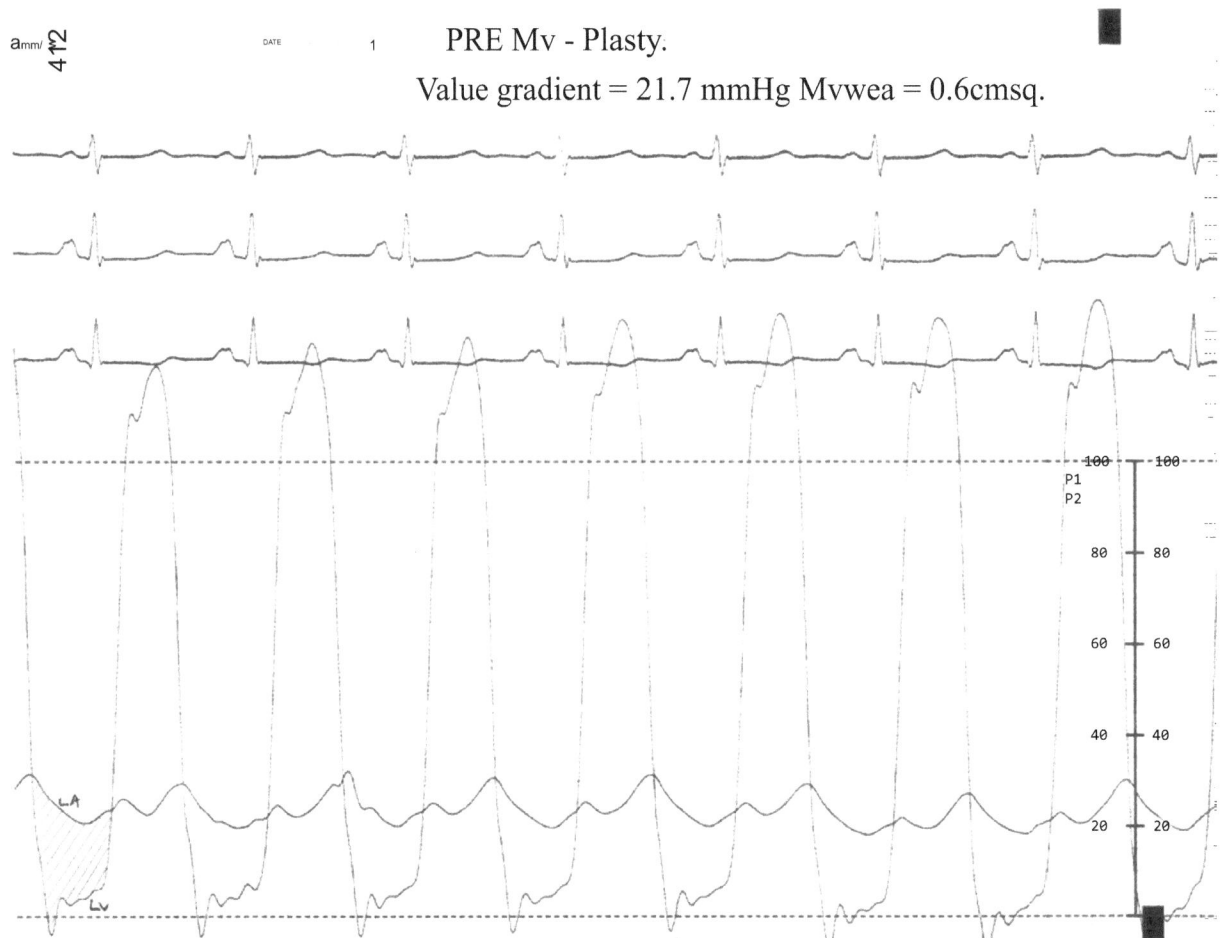

PRE Mv - Plasty.

Value gradient = 21.7 mmHg Mvwea = 0.6cmsq.

Figure 8: Simultaneous left atrial pressure (LA) and left ventricular pressure (LV) for a patient pre-PBMV on the same 100 mm Hg range scale. The area between the curves (shaded) represents the mean transmitral pressure which, in this patient is calculated at 21.7mmHg. The mitral valve area (MVA) was calculated at 0.6cm^2 in this patient (Gorlin's equation).

Once you have advanced the transspetal sheath over the needle into the left atrium, you should removed the obturator and needle from the sheath. At this point the sheath should be carefully de-aired and flushed and heparin can be administered at 80-100 iu/Kg. Simultaneous left atrial and ventricular pressure will give you the instantaneous trans-mitral pressure gradient with a mean gradient calculated as the area between the curves (Figs. **8** and **9**). The Gorlin's equation may also be used to calculate the mitral valve area.

50mm/s   DATE   Post 2ⁿᵈInflation

MVA = 1.6 cmsq MV grad = 7.6 mmHg

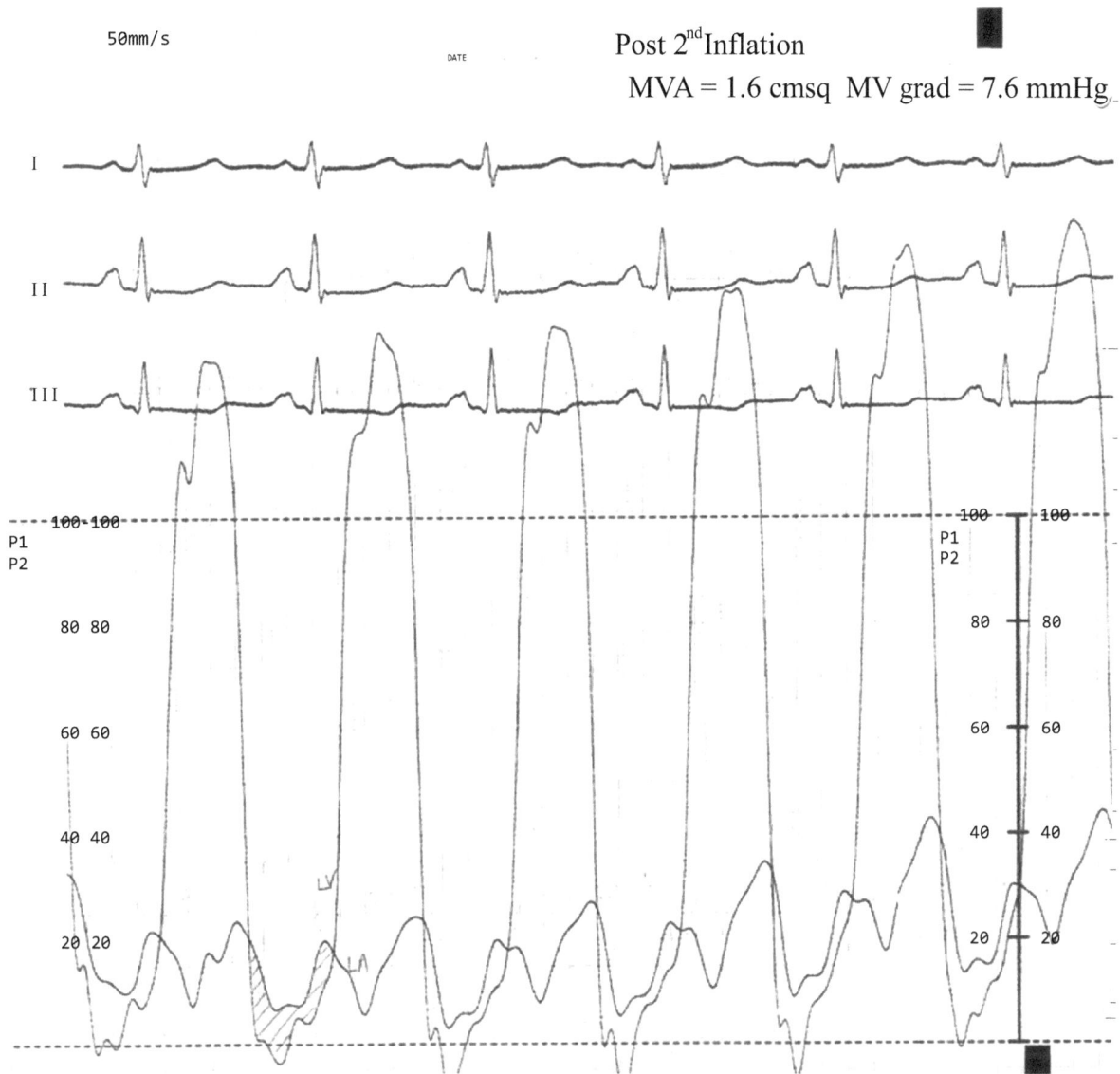

Figure 9: Simultaneous left atrial pressure (LA) and left ventricular pressure (LV) for the same patient as Fig. **8** after two balloon inflations. The area between the curves (shaded) represents the mean transmitral pressure which, post-procedure was calculated at 7.6 mmHg. The mitral valve area (MVA) was calculated at 1.6cm^2 (Gorlin's equation). Note that the reduction in gradient is predominately due to a reduction in left atrial pressure.

The "curly" Inoue guidewire is then placed into the left atrium *via* the transseptal sheath until it is coiled at least twice around the enlarged left atrium (Fig. **10a**). This strong steel wire gives excellent support and stability in the left atrium. The transeptal sheath is then removed and the atrial septal puncture is dilated with the black 14F dilator. Patients often find the atrial stretching painful and it is worth pre-empting this with analgesia.

Patient height and transthoracic echocardiographic measurement should be used determined the optimal stretch diameter and therefore Inoue balloon. Dilute contract (one fifth strength) is used to flush the Inoue Balloon Catheter (IBC) *via* the "vent tube" until it is seen to come out of the main stopcock. The inner tube should be flushed with heparinised saline.

You should start with a conservative stretch diameter as the valvuloplasty can be repeated several times assuming there are no complications. Fill the syringe supplied with the IBC with contrast to the marker appropriate to your selected stretch diameter. You should test that the syringe yields the desired stretch diameter outside the body using the callipers supplied.

Next the balloon of the IBC is stretched by inserting the "inner tube" into the "slot" of the IBC and tightening it. This generates a lower profile for passing the IBC through the skin and the atrial septum over the "curly" Inoue guidewire. Once the IBC is in the left atrium you should release the "inner tube" from the IBC "slot" which allows the IBC tip to bend and follow the line of the "curly" Inoue guidewire (Fig. **10b**). Injecting a little contract into the IBC helps to prevents it falling back into the right atrium (Fig. **10b**).

Once the IBC is stable in the left atrium and pointing inferiorly (Fig. **10b**) you can remove the "curly" Inoue guidewire. In its place insert the stylet. This is not a guidwire and is used to manoeuvre the IBC through the mitral orifice and down to the left ventricular apex. This is achieved by a complex of simultaneous three-dimension movements.

Pull back the IBC until it starts to point down to the MV (you will see it move on the valve and use the stored venticulogram as a road map). The action to locate the correct position involves withdrawing the IBC whilst at the same time anti-clockwise torquing the stylet. Once in position, whilst maintaining the stylet torque, withdraw the stylet 1-2cm and at the same time advance the IBC a little. The IBC should jump forward into the left ventricle.

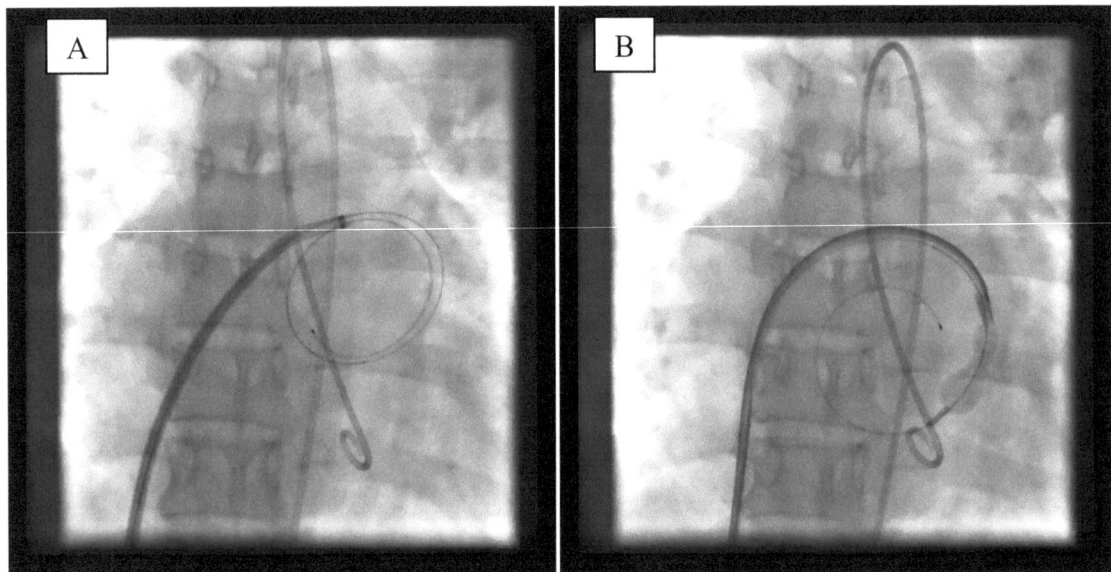

Figure 10: A) Transseptal sheath and "curly" Inoue guidewire are both seen in the left atrium. B) The Inoue balloon catheter is passed over the "curly" Inoue guidewire into the left atrium. (no fluoroscopy angulation).

Always pass the IBC to the left ventricular apex. If you are unable to do so then it is likely that the IBC is caught in the mitral subvalvular apparatus. Inflating the IBC in this position risks avulsing the papillary muscles and must not been attempted. Instead gently withdraw the IBC back into left atrium and recross the mitral valve using the same technique.

Once you are satisfied with the IBC position, inject enough contrast into the IBC to inflate the distal balloon fully. Pull the IBC back until it lodges on the mitral valve (Fig. **11a**) and briskly fully inflate the balloon until the waist disappears (Figs. **11b-d**). Once this is completed briskly deflate the IBC and withdraw it back into the left atrium (the IBC is usually ejected into the left atrium by ventricular systole). If you are unable to get the IBC to lodge in the mitral valve orifice long enough to fully inflate, then either the stretch diameter is too small or the valve is less stenosed than the measurements suggest.

After each valvuloplasty reassess the valve gradient, mitral valve area and the degree of regurgitation using echocardiography and catheter measurements. Success of the procedure is judged by a reduction in the trans-mitral gradient and commissural splitting resulting in increased mitral valve orifice area. Mitral valve orifice area should be confirmed by planimetry (echocardiography) as the pressure half time method may be inaccurate in the acute setting [171]. If there has been a significant decrease in trans-mitral gradient or increase in mitral valve area the procedure should be stopped. If there has been no significant improvement, in the absence of moderate or severe mitral regurgitation, the dilation can be repeated, increasing by 1 or 2mm increments. Using this stepwise dilatation technique and checking for mitral regurgitation in between dilatations is important for achieving functionally significant dilatation whilst minimizing the risk of harm.

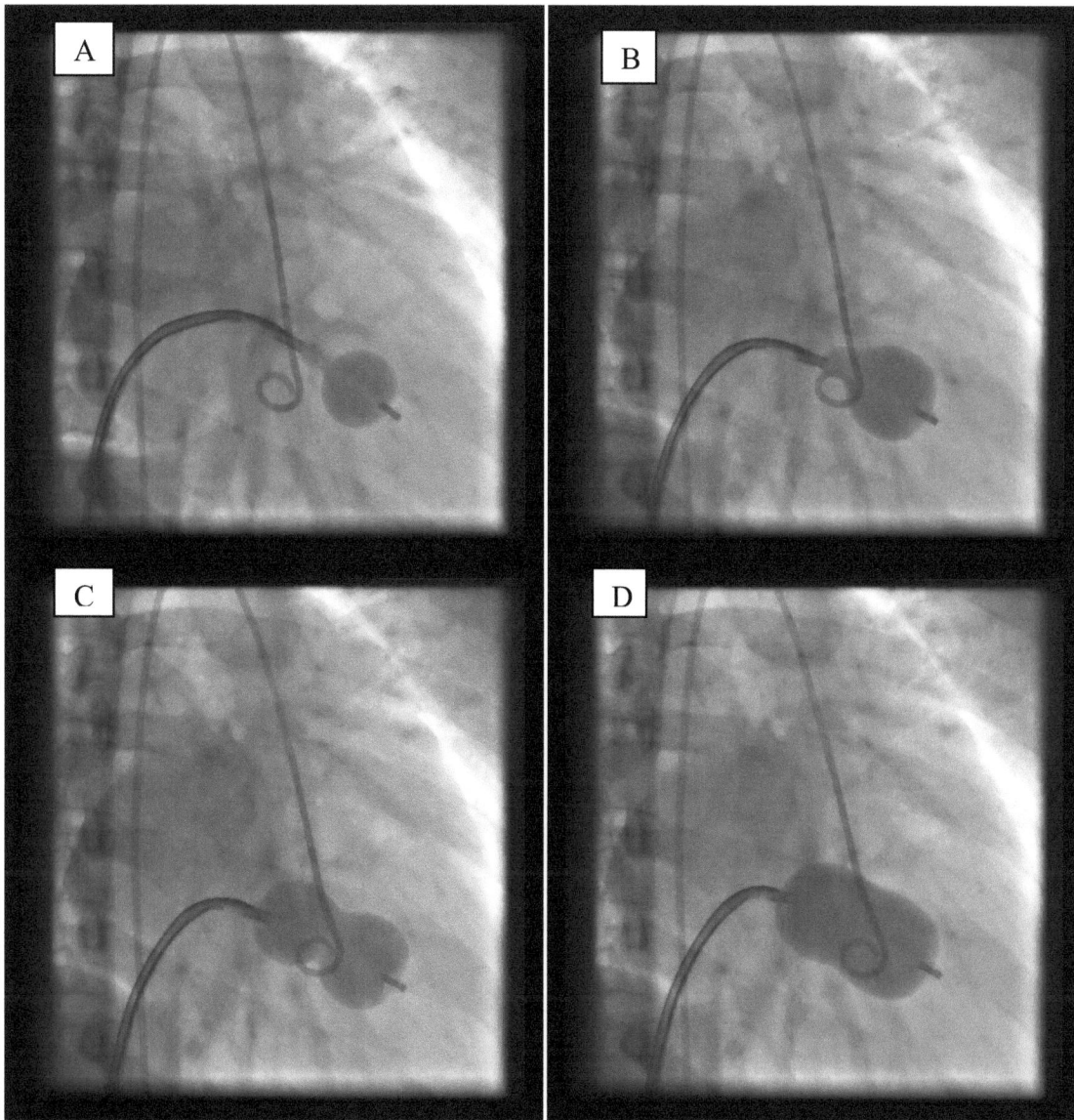

Figure 11: (A & B) Distal balloon is inflated and withdrawn until resistance is felt. (C) Inflation of proximal balloon secures balloon in mitral valve orifice. (D) Inflation of middle section of balloon causes dilatation of mitral valve (balloon waist can be seen to disappear).

Complications of Inoue PBMV

Complications from PBMV are rare when it is performed by experienced operators in carefully selected patients. The three main complications of Inoue PBMV are haemopericardium (potentially leading to tamponade), systemic embolism (usually cerebrovascular event) and severe mitral regurgitation. Haemopericardium is usually due to inadvertent puncture of structures adjacent to the septum by the Brockenbough needle during the transseptal puncture, but can also rarely be caused by perforation of the left atrium or left ventricular apex by the guidewire or balloon. The incidence of haemopericardium is listed at 0.6%-0.9% in large series that used the Inoue technique exclusively.

Systemic embolism is a rare but potentially devastating complication and usually manifests as a cerebrovascular event. It is usually caused by thrombotic material but can be caused by disruption of calcification. Transoesophageal echocardiography should be performed prior to the procedure to exclude the presence of left atrial thrombus [172].

Systemic embolisation is reported at an incidence of 0.5%-0.9% in series that use the IBC exclusively, and as high as 1.8% in series that contain other PBMV techniques [149].

Severe mitral regurgitation occurs in 1.4%-6% of the selected Inoue series, and 9.4% in a mixed Inoue and double balloon PBMV series (149). It is usually caused by non commissural tearing of the leaflets and had been shown to be predicted by the presence of severe calcification of the mitral valve [165].

Atrial septal defect is a common finding after PMBV if it is looked for (up to 62%) of patients, however the majority of these are seen to decrease in size over time and they are very rarely haemodynamically significant [173]. Some defects have been caused by premature inflation of cylindrical balloons, or withdrawal of winged balloons. These complications seem to be less frequent with the Inoue balloon [174].

Mortality from the procedure ranges from 0% to 0.5%, and urgent surgery is required in 1.2% [175]. Indications for urgent surgery are haemopericardium unresponsive to pericardiocentesis, or urgent mitral valve replacement because of haemodynamic compromise secondary to severe mitral regurgitation.

Table 2: Complications recorded in series containing patients undergoing PBMV *via* the Inoue technique and a combination of the Inoue and double balloon PBMV technique. Chen *et al.* [176], Hernandez et a [175], Neumayer *et al.* [177], Fawzy *et al.* [3], Palacious *et al.* [149], Ing *et al.* [178].

Study	Death %	Severe MR %	Embolic event %	Tamponade %
Studies containing Inoue technique only				
Chen *et al.*	0.1	1.4	0.5	0.8
Hernandez *et al.*	0.5	4.0	-	0.6
Neumayer *et al.*	0.4	6.0	0.9	0.9
Fawzy *et al.*	0	1.8	0.6	0.8
Studies containg Inoue and double balloon technique				
Palacious *et al.*	0.6	9.4	1.8	1.0
Iung *et al.*	0.4	4.1	0.4	0.2

Short and Long Term Results

Procedural success is usually defined as a final valve area $>1.5cm^2$ in the absence of moderate or severe mitral regurgitation. Success rates in large series (which usually feature younger patients with favourable valve morphology) approaches 100%, with a doubling of mitral valve area post procedure not uncommon.

Randomised controlled trials indicates that results are at least as favourable for PBMV as they are for open commissurotomy in the short and intermediate term, up to 7 years [179, 180]. However, it should be remembered that both these trials only included patients with favourable valve morphology and while PBMV is the first choice treatment for patients with favourable valve anatomy, open commissurotomy, or more commonly in recent practice mitral valve replacement remain valuable treatment options for patients with unfavourable valve anatomy.

Long-term follow up data is now available for PBMV and event free survival (defined as survival without death, repeat PBMV, mitral valve replacement or NHYA class III or IV) is as high as 74% at 13 years (3). PBMV has also been shown to have a beneficial effect on exercise capacity [181] and to produce a gradual decrease in pulmonary artery pressure and pulmonary vascular resistance [182]. Independent predictors of poor late results were low valve area and high gradient immediately following PBMV, old age, unfavourable valve anatomy, high NYHA class pre-procedure, atrial fibrillation and mitral regurgitation greater than 2/4 post-PBMV [183].

Other Techniques for PBMV

Techniques other than the Inoue technique have been described for PBMV and have been used successfully. Shortly after the first PBMC using the Inoue balloon was described, Lock *et al.* described the use of a cylindrical balloon

[184]. However, this often resulted in inadequate dilatation and was replaced with a method involving double balloons [185]. Along with the Inoue technique, the double balloon technique is one of the two main methods of PBMV currently in use. It is more complicated than the Inoue technique involving the use of two guidewires and two balloons being positioned in the mitral valve. This leads to longer procedural times. A multi–track system has been developed that uses a monorail system requiring only one guidewire but it is not in widespread use [186]. A prospective randomised controlled trial between Inoue and double balloon valvotomy showed no significant differences in immediate results or complications [187]. Procedural difficulties were more commonly encountered in the double balloon method [188], and a higher risk of ventricular apical perforation was reported [189].

Table 3: Immediate and long term results of series containing patients undergoing PBMV *via* the Inoue technique and a combination of the Inoue and double balloon PBMV technique. MVA (mitral valve area). Chen *et al.* [173], Hernandez *et al.* [175], Neumayer *et al.* [177], Fawzy *et al.* [3], Palacious *et al.* [149], Ing *et al.* [178].

Immediate results			Late results	
Studies containing Inoue technique only				
	Pre MVA cm^2	Post MVA cm^2	Follow up (yrs)	Event free survival%
Chen *et al.*	1.1	2.1	-	-
Hernandez *et al.*	1.0	1.8	7	69
Neumayer *et al.*	1.1	1.8	-	-
Fawzy *et al.*	0.9	2.0	13	74
Studies containing Inoue and double balloon technique				
Palacious *et al.*	0.9	1.9	12	33
Iung *et al.*	1.0	1.9	10	56

A technique involving a metallic commissurotome has been described by Cribier *et al.* [190] with results comparable to balloon valvuloplasty. The technique is more demanding on the operator than the Inoue technique and carries a theoretical higher chance of haemopericardium due to the stiffer guide wire. However as the commissurotome can be sterilized for multiple use, it may represent a cost effective solution for developing countries where rheumatic heart disease is endemic.

Special Cases

Congenital Mitral Stenosis

PBMV seems attractive in severe congenital mitral stenosis as it obviates the requirement for thoracotomy. Unfortunately in a review of children undergoing PBMV and surgery for mitral stenosis due to typical congenital MS the results have been disappointing [191]. This study included patients with thickened leaflets, short or absent chordae tendineae, obliteration of interchordal spaces, two separate but often closely spaced papillary muscles, parachute mitral valve, supravalvular mitral ring and double-orifice mitral valve. Surgical resection was preferable for a supra-valvular ring. For patients undergoing PBMV, survival free from re-intervention (for restenosis or because of mitral regurgitation) was only 55% at 5 years [191].

Pregnancy

Mitral stenosis is more prevalent in women than men (2:1) and its presence is often unmasked by the haemodynamic changes and increase in intra-vascular volume that occurs with pregnancy. Maternal mortality for patients in NYHA class 1 or 2 is low 0.4% and can potentially be managed medically. It is significantly higher for those in NYHA 3 or 4 (6.8%) [192] and PBMV may be considered after the first trimester. This has been shown to feasible with abdominal shielding [193] and has also been performed with echocardiography rather than fluoroscopy guidance [194].

Older Patients with Unfavourable Anatomy

In developed countries it is becoming increasingly common for patients to present at much older ages. They often have a calcified, immobile valve with significant sub-valvular disease. In these patients surgery would be the treatment option of choice, however, they often have considerable co-morbidities that make them poor surgical candidates. PBMV has been shown to be an effective therapy in patients >65 years of age [195] and can provide some palliation of symptoms in patients with unfavourable valve anatomy although it has to be accepted that immediate increase in valve area and long term results will not be as favourable as in patients undergoing the procedure with favourable valve anatomy [196].

PULMONARY STENOSIS

Pathophysiology

Pulmonary stenosis can be defined as an anatomic obstruction to blood flow from the right ventricular outflow tract to the pulmonary artery. The outflow obstruction is usually located at the level of the pulmonary valve, but may also be supra-valvular or sub-valvular, when it will often occur in association with other congenital cardiac abnormalities. Valvular pulmonary stenosis is usually congenital in aetiology [197]. Acquired causes are considerably less common and include rheumatic fever and carcinoid syndrome. Rarely, the valve apparatus may also be compressed extrinsically by cardiac tumours or aneurysms of the sinus of valsalva. This chapter will only focus on true valvular pulmonary stenosis.

Stenosis of the pulmonary valve is one of the more common manifestations of congenital heart disease, constituting 7.5% to 9.0% of all congenital heart defects [198] As an isolated abnormality, it occurs in approximately 7.0 / 10000 live births [199]. There are three main abnormal valve morphologies of clinical significance.

1.   The classical dome-shaped valve is characterized by a narrow central opening with fused leaflets but a preserved, mobile valve mechanism. Clearly defined commissures may not be identifiable, although three rudimentary raphes are usually seen. Post-stenotic dilatation of the pulmonary outflow tract is usually present.

2.   The dysplastic valve occurs in approximately 20% of patients with valvular pulmonary stenosis and is frequent in patients with Noonan's syndrome. The valve leaflets are markedly thickened, nodular, and poorly mobile and there is no commissural fusion. The pulmonary trunk and annulus are often narrowed.

3.   Less common variants include the unicuspid or bicuspid pulmonary valve which may occur in patients with Tetralogy of Fallot.

Patients with pulmonary stenosis can present at any stage from birth to adulthood and may present with a wide spectrum of clinical features, depending on the degree of obstruction and the size of the valve orifice, which may vary from a pinhole to several millimetres in diameter. Neonates with severe obstruction of the pulmonary valve may present with central cyanosis, due to right-to-left shunting at the atrial level and may require prostaglandin infusions to maintain a patent ductus arteriosus thus perfusing the lungs with aortic blood.

Infants and children may be diagnosed after a routine examination which identifies a murmur. Adults with isolated pulmonary stenosis will often remain asymptomatic until severe right ventricular outflow tract obstruction occurs. At this point, symptoms will be those of right ventricular pressure overload – breathlessness, fatigue, light-headedness and angina-like pain which is thought to be attributable to the increased myocardial oxygen demand of the hypertrophied right ventricle.

The diagnosis of pulmonary stenosis will often be suspected by the detection of an ejection systolic murmur at the upper left sternal edge, and may occur in association with a right ventricular heave. The electrocardiogram can show features of right atrial or right ventricular hypertrophy and a chest radiograph may reveal prominent pulmonary artery shadows.

Echocardiography remains the mainstay of diagnosis. Two-dimensional echo may reveal thickened pulmonary valve leaflets, and Doppler interrogation will demonstrate increased transvalvular velocity which can be used to calculate peak and mean pressure gradients. Calculation of the pulmonary valve area using the continuity equation is possible but not well established. Cardiac catheterization is usually not required for the diagnosis of pulmonary stenosis.

Natural History

The natural history of pulmonary stenosis varies depending on the severity of the valve lesion. Most patients with peak instantaneous trans-valvular gradients less than 50 mm Hg [200] or peak right ventricular systolic pressure less than 75 mm Hg [201] are slow to progress beyond these thresholds at follow-up. More severe lesions will often progress with time to greater degrees of stenosis. Furthermore, children under 2 years of age with mild stenosis appear more likely to progress to moderate or severe disease than adult patients with mild stenotic lesions [201, 203].

Current guidelines on the management of pulmonary stenosis reflect what is known about the natural history of the condition. It is recommended that all patients undergo an initial evaluation with clinical examination, electrocardiogram, chest radiograph and two-dimensional echocardiography with Doppler. Patients with a peak instantaneous trans-valvular gradient by Doppler less than 30 mmHg are advised to undergo follow-up assessments at 5-yearly intervals. Those with a peak gradient between 30 and 50 mm Hg should be followed up on an annual basis with routine echocardiographic analysis every 2 to 5 years [1].

For patients with severe, classically domed pulmonary valvular stenosis, percutaneous balloon valvuloplasty is now the treatment of choice. The first catheter attempt at pulmonary valvulotomy was in 1956 by Rubio and Limon Lason [204], who used a ureteral catheter with a wire to cut open a stenosed pulmonary valve. In 1979, Semb *et al.* [205] used a balloon filled with carbon dioxide to pull back across the pulmonary valve in a retrograde manner from the pulmonary artery to the right ventricular outflow tract. Unfortunately, this method was associated with a significant risk of avulsion of the pulmonary valve leaflets. In 1982, Kan *et al.* described the first successful case of percutaneous pulmonary balloon valvuloplasty in an eight year old child with congenital pulmonary valve stenosis, using a static form of dilatation which is still used today [206].

Percutaneous balloon pulmonary valvuloplasty is recommended for asymptomatic patients with a domed pulmonary valve with a peak gradient greater than 60 mm Hg (or mean gradient greater than 40 mm Hg), as well as for symptomatic patients with a peak gradient greater than 50 mm Hg (or mean gradient greater than 30 mm Hg) [207].

Pulmonary valve dysplasia has been implicated by some authors as a predictor of poor procedural success following percutaneous balloon valvuloplasty [208, 209]. However, other groups have reported better success rates [201,210] leading some authors [203] to recommend balloon valvuloplasty as the first line therapy for patients with severe pulmonary stenosis secondary to a dysplastic valve. In keeping with these mixed outcomes the American College of Cardiology / American Heart Association guidelines state that balloon valvotomy "may be reasonable" patients with a dysplastic pulmonary valve, given the same haemodynamic conditions as described above for patients with domed pulmonary valve stenosis [207].

Percutaneous balloon pulmonary valvuloplasty is not recommended for patients with moderate or severe pulmonary regurgitation, subvalvular or supravalvular pulmonary stenosis, or if there is an associated hypoplastic pulmonary annulus. For these patients, and for those with concomitant severe tricuspid regurgitation, current guidelines recommend surgical therapy. [16]

Pulmonary Valvuloplasty - the Procedure

Patients are usually sedated for percutaneous balloon pulmonary valvuloplasty, although the degree of sedation will vary depending on the age of the patient and local practices. Most adult patients will receive oral benzodiazepines prior to the start of the procedure, with supplemental doses of intravenous Midazolam and/or Fentanyl used throughout. Continuous monitoring of blood pressure is usually performed with a femoral arterial sheath in situ, and monitoring of heart rate, respiratory rate, and pulse oximetry is strongly recommended throughout the procedure.

The right femoral vein is the preferred and most commonly used access point, although jugular and axillary veins can also be used if required. The groin should be shaved and appropriately cleaned and draped to provide an aseptic field. Using the Seldinger technique, a small (4-6 French) sheath should be inserted into the femoral vein. A multipurpose catheter can then be introduced into the femoral sheath and advanced into the right ventricle under fluoroscopic guidance. At this point, a right ventriculogram can be obtained with the catheter positioned in the RV outflow tract to increase the likelihood of detecting a pinhole opening through the valve.

Crossing the pulmonary valve can be attempted with one of a number of preformed catheters, including Judkins right, balloon wedge, or angled glidecath catheters. Often, however, it will not be possible to advance a catheter directly through a critically narrowed pulmonary valve such that a soft-tipped guide wire may be necessary. Once the valve has been crossed by the selected catheter, a 0.014 inch to 0.035 inch J-tipped, exchange-length, guidewire can be carefully advanced into the left or right pulmonary arteries.

Haemodynamic assessment of the severity of pulmonary stenosis should be attempted with measurement of right ventricular (second pigtail catheter) and pulmonary artery pressures along with peak-to-peak transvalvular gradients. A right ventricular peak systolic pressure greater than 75% of peak systolic systemic pressure (as measured by simultaneous recording taken from the femoral artery) is considered a useful marker of severity of obstruction across the pulmonary valve [207].

A number of balloons are available in the UK, including the Cristal Balloon (Pyramed Ltd, UK) and the Z-Med™ Balloon (NuMED Inc, Hopkinton NY). Balloons come in various sizes and are actually quite compliant with a broad range of size depending on the pressure generated by the indeflator or syringe. This makes accurate sizing of the balloon difficult. The large volume required to fill the balloon and the rapidity at which inflation must occur, means that a specialized indeflator such as those used in transcatheter aortic valve implantation procedures or a 30ml syringe must be used.

Balloon diameter is an important technical factor that needs to be taken into account when considering the strategy behind percutaneous balloon pulmonary valvuloplasty. Current guidelines recommend the use of balloons that are 1.2 – 1.4 times the diameter of the pulmonary valve annulus [16]. This is based on data from studies which demonstrated significantly fewer immediate suboptimal outcomes [211] and follow-up restenosis rates [212] when compared with balloon : annulus ratios less than 1.2. Balloons greater than 1.4 times the annulus diameter have been associated with higher rates of pulmonary regurgitation at long-term follow-up [213].

Furthermore, those with balloon : annulus ratios greater than 1.5 have not been found to produce superior results to balloons that are 1.2 to 1.5 times the annulus diameter [212] and in theory, may be more likely to damage the right ventricular outflow tract. As such, balloon : annulus ratios of 1.4 to 1.5 are not recommended for patients with classical doming pulmonary stenosis, although some authors have suggested that they may be beneficial for patients with dysplastic valve morphology [198]. For those patients with a very large pulmonary valve annulus, particularly adults, it may be preferable to perform valvuloplasty with the simultaneous inflation of two balloons across the pulmonary valve. However, this technique has not been shown to produce superior results to a single balloon technique [203].

Outcome

Percutaneous balloon pulmonary valvuloplasty is a safe procedure with a low incidence of acute complications. In the Valvuloplasty and Angioplasty of Congenital Anomalies (VACA) registry reporting on 822 procedures performed in 26 institutions, there were 5 reported major complications (0.6%), including two deaths (0.2%) and one cardiac perforation with tamponade (0.1%) [214]. The incidence of major and minor complications was significantly higher in neonates and infants than in adults. Transient bradycardia, catheter-induced ventricular ectopy and a decrease in systemic blood pressure during balloon inflation are common, and almost always return to normal following balloon deflation. Other serious complications are rare but include complete heart block, tricuspid valve papillary muscle rupture, pulmonary artery tears, pulmonary oedema, requirement for surgical intervention and cardiac arrest [215].

Numerous studies have reported on the favourable results after percutaneous balloon valvuloplasty for congenital pulmonary stenosis. Consistent findings immediately after the procedure include statistically significant reductions in right ventricular systolic pressure, and a reduction in right ventricle to pulmonary artery peak systolic pressure gradients [4, 216, 217].

A suboptimal immediate outcome, defined in most series as a residual catheter gradient greater than 30 – 35 mm Hg, is uncommon and occurs in 4.8 to 6% of patients [4, 216]. In the series by Jarrar *et al.*, of those patients with an immediate suboptimal outcome, two-thirds had dysplastic valvular morphology, but all three patients had unchanged gradients at repeat catheterisation four to six years after the initial procedure (4). In contrast to these results, Fawzy *et al.* found that all five patients with suboptimal outcomes developed restenosis at six to twelve months after balloon valvuloplasty and attributed that to the use of small balloon catheters early in their experience. All five patients subsequently went on to have successful repeat valvuloplasty with larger balloons [216].

Excellent results are also generally maintained at intermediate and long-term follow-up. Within the first two years of follow-up, rates of true restenosis (*i.e.* after an acceptable immediate reduction in peak pulmonary gradient) vary between 4.8 and 11% [4,218]. Long-term outcomes (*i.e.* 10 to 17 years after the initial procedure) reveal a minimal (1 – 2%) late recurrence of pulmonary stenosis (beyond what was seen at intermediate-term follow-up). Rates of pulmonary regurgitation vary from 39% [4] to 90% [218], and the prevalence appears to increase with time. However, the vast majority of cases are mild in severity and rarely of haemodynamic significance, with most series reporting no cases of right ventricular volume overload or need for surgical intervention [216, 218].

Predictors of Long-term Results

In the large Valvuloplasty and Angioplasty of Congenital Anomalies (VACA) registry, follow-up data was available on 533 patients for a mean of 8.7 years after balloon pulmonary valvuloplasty. In that study, the most significant independent predictors of long-term results were valve morphology, valve hinge point diameter, balloon to valve dimension ratio and immediate haemodynamic results [213]. Most studies have reported an increased frequency of suboptimal results following balloon dilatation of dysplastic pulmonary valves, although Rao did demonstrated improved results in these patients with the use of oversized balloons (balloon : annulus ratio 1.4-1.5) [198].

Balloon pulmonary valvuloplasty appears to act by splitting fused commissures and this feature is probably absent in severely dysplastic valves. However, it is clear that varying degrees of valve dysplasia occur in patients with pulmonary stenosis and this may explain the discrepancy in results obtained from balloon dilatation of these valves. Guidelines reflect this uncertainty, with percutaneous balloon valvuloplasty having a class IIb indication for the management of patients with dysplastic pulmonary valves[1].

For patients with classical "doming" pulmonary stenosis, immediate post-valvuloplasty gradient greater than 30 mm Hg and a balloon : pulmonary valve annulus ratio less than 1.2 have been associated with a higher probability of restenosis, and a ratio greater than 1.4 with a significantly increased incidence of important pulmonary regurgitation [213]. As such, optimal results appear to be achieved with balloon : annulus ratios between 1.2 and 1.4.

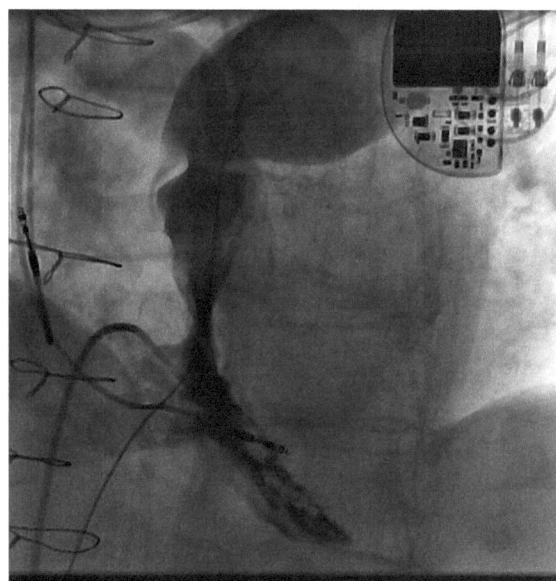

Figure 12: Right ventriculogram demonstrating pulmonary stenosis (arrow) with marked post-stenotic dilatation of the pulmonary trunk (no fluoroscopic angulation).

Comparison of Pulmonary Valvuloplasty with Surgery

Before the development of balloon pulmonary valvuloplasty, surgical treatment was the only definitive management option for valvular pulmonary stenosis. As such, long-term follow-up data is available for patients who have undergone a surgical approach, but comparison with balloon valvuloplasty is difficult to interpret because of inherent problems in comparing older surgical techniques with newer percutaneous therapies. In addition, there are fewer numbers and a relatively shorter duration of available follow-up data for patients who have undergone balloon valvuloplasty.

Notwithstanding these limitations, balloon pulmonary valvuloplasty has been shown to have a number of clear advantages over surgical treatment. Procedural mortality is significantly lower with the percutaneous balloon approach (0.2% versus 3 – 14%), as is the incidence and severity of pulmonary regurgitation at long-term follow-up [212]. In fact, in a recent series of 53 surgical patients, 70% were noted to have moderate to severe pulmonary regurgitation at long-term follow-up (18 – 51 years, mean 33 years), and 21 (40%) had required re-intervention with a pulmonary valve replacement [219]. Although, early comparisons did demonstrate higher recurrences of pulmonary stenosis with balloon valvuloplasty versus surgery (14-23% vs. 0-8%), these results occurred at a time when small balloons (balloon : annulus ratios less than 1.0) were used [220] It should be noted that Rao *et al.* observed no recurrences with the use of balloons larger than 1.2 times the valve annulus [212].

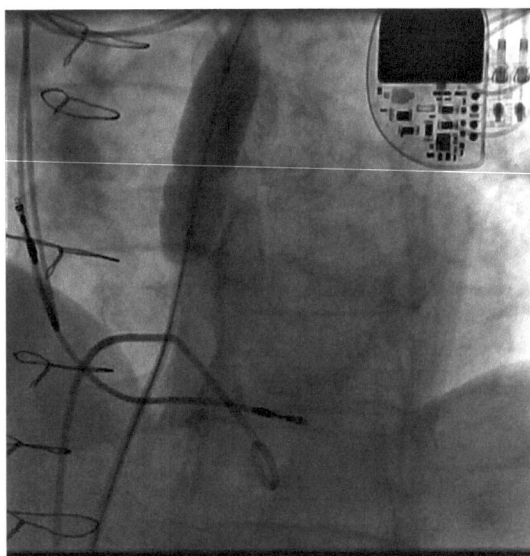

Figure 13: Valvuloplasty of pulmonary stenosis in the same patient with similar projection as Fig. 13. The balloon is seen to "waist" at the level of the pulmonary valve (arrow) (no fluoroscopic angulation).

REFERENCES

[1]   Warnes CA, Williams RG, Bashore TM, Child JS, Connolly HM, Dearani JA, *et al.* ACC/AHA 2008 Guidelines for the Management of Adults with Congenital Heart Disease: a report of the American College of Cardiology/American Heart Association Task Force on Practice Guidelines (writing committee to develop guidelines on the management of adults with congenital heart disease). Circulation 2008; 118(23): e714-833.

[2]   Moore P, Egito E, Mowrey H, Perry SB, Lock JE, Keane JF. Midterm results of balloon dilation of congenital aortic stenosis: predictors of success. J Am Coll Cardiol 1996; 27(5): 1257-63.

[3]   Fawzy ME, Hegazy H, Shoukri M, El Shaer F, ElDali A, Al-Amri M. Long-term clinical and echocardiographic results after successful mitral balloon valvotomy and predictors of long-term outcome. Eur Heart J 2005; 26(16): 1647-52.

[4]   Jarrar M, Betbout F, Farhat MB, Maatouk F, Gamra H, Addad F, *et al.* Long-term invasive and noninvasive results of percutaneous balloon pulmonary valvuloplasty in children, adolescents, and adults. Am Heart J 1999; 138(5 Pt 1): 950-4.

[5]   Bonow RO, Carabello BA, Chatterjee K, de Leon AC, Jr., Faxon DP, Freed MD, *et al.* 2008 Focused update incorporated into the ACC/AHA 2006 guidelines for the management of patients with valvular heart disease: a report of the American College of Cardiology/American Heart Association Task Force on Practice Guidelines (Writing Committee to Revise the 1998 Guidelines for the Management of Patients With Valvular Heart Disease): endorsed by the Society of Cardiovascular

Anesthesiologists, Society for Cardiovascular Angiography and Interventions, and Society of Thoracic Surgeons. Circulation 2008; 118(15): e523-661.

[6]   Aboulhosn J, Child JS. Left ventricular outflow obstruction: subaortic stenosis, bicuspid aortic valve, supravalvar aortic stenosis, and coarctation of the aorta. Circulation 2006; 114(22): 2412-22.

[7]   Duran AC, Frescura C, Sans-Coma V, Angelini A, Basso C, Thiene G. Bicuspid aortic valves in hearts with other congenital heart disease. J Heart Valve Dis 1995; 4(6): 581-90.

[8]   Mack G, Silberbach M. Aortic and pulmonary stenosis. Pediatr Rev 2000; 21(3): 79-85.

[9]   Gershoni-Baruch R, Moor EV, Enat R. Marfan syndrome associated with bicuspid aortic valve, premature aging, and primary hypogonadism. Am J Med Genet 1990; 37(2): 169-72.

[10]   Petitalot JP, Chaix AF, Rousseau G, Barraine R. [Marfan's or Marfan-like syndrome: value of echocardiography]. Rev Med Interne 1987; 8(1): 27-36.

[11]   Emanuelsson H, Olsson SB. [Balloon dilatation of aortic valve stenosis--an alternative to surgery]. Lakartidningen 1987; 84(20): 1756.

[12]   Porciani MC, Attanasio M, Lepri V, Lapini I, Demarchi G, Padeletti L, *et al.* [Prevalence of cardiovascular manifestations in Marfan syndrome]. Ital Heart J Suppl 2004; 5(8): 647-52.

[13]   Hirose H, Amano A, Takahashi A, Nagano N, Kohmoto T. Ruptured aortic dissecting aneurysm in Turner's syndrome: a case report and review of literature. Ann Thorac Cardiovasc Surg 2000; 6(4): 275-80.

[14]   De Mozzi P, Longo UG, Galanti G, Maffulli N. Bicuspid aortic valve: a literature review and its impact on sport activity. Br Med Bull 2008; 85: 63-85.

[15]   Vallely MP, Semsarian C, Bannon PG. Management of the ascending aorta in patients with bicuspid aortic valve disease. Heart Lung Circ 2008; 17(5): 357-63.

[16]   Roberts WC. The congenitally bicuspid aortic valve. A study of 85 autopsy cases. Am J Cardiol 1970; 26(1): 72-83.

[17]   Roberts WC, Ko JM. Frequency by decades of unicuspid, bicuspid, and tricuspid aortic valves in adults having isolated aortic valve replacement for aortic stenosis, with or without associated aortic regurgitation. Circulation 2005; 111(7): 920-5.

[18]   Roberts WC, Morrow AG, McIntosh CL, Jones M, Epstein SE. Congenitally bicuspid aortic valve causing severe, pure aortic regurgitation without superimposed infective endocarditis. Analysis of 13 patients requiring aortic valve replacement. Am J Cardiol 1981; 47(2): 206-9.

[19]   Beppu S, Suzuki S, Matsuda H, Ohmori F, Nagata S, Miyatake K. Rapidity of progression of aortic stenosis in patients with congenital bicuspid aortic valves. Am J Cardiol 1993; 71(4): 322-7.

[20]   Fedak PW, Verma S, David TE, Leask RL, Weisel RD, Butany J. Clinical and pathophysiological implications of a bicuspid aortic valve. Circulation 2002; 106(8): 900-4.

[21]   Tadros TM, Klein MD, Shapira OM. Ascending aortic dilatation associated with bicuspid aortic valve: pathophysiology, molecular biology, and clinical implications. Circulation 2009; 119(6): 880-90.

[22]   Sadler TW. Langman's Medical Embryology. 6th ed. Balitmore: William's and Wilkins; 1990.

[23]   Kappetein AP, Gittenberger-de Groot AC, Zwinderman AH, Rohmer J, Poelmann RE, Huysmans HA. The neural crest as a possible pathogenetic factor in coarctation of the aorta and bicuspid aortic valve. J Thorac Cardiovasc Surg 1991; 102(6): 830-6.

[24]   Kirby ML, Waldo KL. Role of neural crest in congenital heart disease. Circulation 1990; 82(2): 332-40.

[25]   Ausoni S, Sartore S. Cell lineages and tissue boundaries in cardiac arterial and venous poles: developmental patterns, animal models, and implications for congenital vascular diseases. Arterioscler Thromb Vasc Biol 2001; 21(3): 312-20.

[26]   Morrison-Graham K, Schatteman GC, Bork T, Bowen-Pope DF, Weston JA. A PDGF receptor mutation in the mouse (Patch) perturbs the development of a non-neuronal subset of neural crest-derived cells. Development 1992; 115(1): 133-42.

[27]   Gulyasy B, Lopez-Candales A, Reis SE, Levitsky S. Quadricuspid aortic valve: an unusual echocardiographic finding and a review of the literature. Int J Cardiol 2009; 132(2): e68-71.

[28]   Huntington K, Hunter AG, Chan KL. A prospective study to assess the frequency of familial clustering of congenital bicuspid aortic valve. J Am Coll Cardiol 1997; 30(7): 1809-12.

[29]   Clementi M, Notari L, Borghi A, Tenconi R. Familial congenital bicuspid aortic valve: a disorder of uncertain inheritance. Am J Med Genet 1996; 62(4): 336-8.

[30]   Miller MJ, Geffner ME, Lippe BM, Itami RM, Kaplan SA, DiSessa TG, *et al.* Echocardiography reveals a high incidence of bicuspid aortic valve in Turner syndrome. J Pediatr 1983; 102(1): 47-50.

[31]   Tutar E, Ekici F, Atalay S, Nacar N. The prevalence of bicuspid aortic valve in newborns by echocardiographic screening. Am Heart J 2005; 150(3): 513-5.

[32]   Basso C, Boschello M, Perrone C, Mecenero A, Cera A, Bicego D, *et al.* An echocardiographic survey of primary school children for bicuspid aortic valve. Am J Cardiol 2004; 93(5): 661-3.

[33] Martin LJ, Ramachandran V, Cripe LH, Hinton RB, Andelfinger G, Tabangin M, *et al.* Evidence in favor of linkage to human chromosomal regions 18q, 5q and 13q for bicuspid aortic valve and associated cardiovascular malformations. Hum Genet 2007; 121(2): 275-84.

[34] Garg V, Muth AN, Ransom JF, Schluterman MK, Barnes R, King IN, *et al.* Mutations in NOTCH1 cause aortic valve disease. Nature 2005; 437(7056): 270-4.

[35] Mohamed SA, Aherrahrou Z, Liptau H, Erasmi AW, Hagemann C, Wrobel S, *et al.* Novel missense mutations (p.T596M and p.P1797H) in NOTCH1 in patients with bicuspid aortic valve. Biochem Biophys Res Commun 2006; 345(4): 1460-5.

[36] Mohamed SA, Hanke T, Schlueter C, Bullerdiek J, Sievers HH. Ubiquitin fusion degradation 1-like gene dysregulation in bicuspid aortic valve. J Thorac Cardiovasc Surg 2005; 130(6): 1531-6.

[37] Ben-Shachar S, Ou Z, Shaw CA, Belmont JW, Patel MS, Hummel M, *et al.* 22q11.2 distal deletion: a recurrent genomic disorder distinct from DiGeorge syndrome and velocardiofacial syndrome. Am J Hum Genet 2008; 82(1): 214-21.

[38] Guo DC, Pannu H, Tran-Fadulu V, Papke CL, Yu RK, Avidan N, *et al.* Mutations in smooth muscle alpha-actin (ACTA2) lead to thoracic aortic aneurysms and dissections. Nat Genet 2007; 39(12): 1488-93.

[39] Aicher D, Urbich C, Zeiher A, Dimmeler S, Schafers HJ. Endothelial nitric oxide synthase in bicuspid aortic valve disease. Ann Thorac Surg 2007; 83(4): 1290-4.

[40] Lee TC, Zhao YD, Courtman DW, Stewart DJ. Abnormal aortic valve development in mice lacking endothelial nitric oxide synthase. Circulation 2000; 101(20): 2345-8.

[41] Ward C. Clinical significance of the bicuspid aortic valve. Heart 2000; 83(1): 81-5.

[42] Grande KJ, Cochran RP, Reinhall PG, Kunzelman KS. Stress variations in the human aortic root and valve: the role of anatomic asymmetry. Ann Biomed Eng 1998; 26(4): 534-45.

[43] Richards KE, Deserranno D, Donal E, Greenberg NL, Thomas JD, Garcia MJ. Influence of structural geometry on the severity of bicuspid aortic stenosis. Am J Physiol Heart Circ Physiol 2004; 287(3): H1410-6.

[44] Robicsek F, Thubrikar MJ, Cook JW, Fowler B. The congenitally bicuspid aortic valve: how does it function? Why does it fail? Ann Thorac Surg 2004; 77(1): 177-85.

[45] Verma S, Szmitko PE, Fedak PW, Errett L, Latter DA, David TE. Can statin therapy alter the natural history of bicuspid aortic valves? Am J Physiol Heart Circ Physiol 2005; 288(6): H2547-9.

[46] Pohle K, Maffert R, Ropers D, Moshage W, Stilianakis N, Daniel WG, *et al.* Progression of aortic valve calcification: association with coronary atherosclerosis and cardiovascular risk factors. Circulation 2001; 104(16): 1927-32.

[47] Demer LL. Cholesterol in vascular and valvular calcification. Circulation 2001; 104(16): 1881-3.

[48] Mohler ER, 3rd, Gannon F, Reynolds C, Zimmerman R, Keane MG, Kaplan FS. Bone formation and inflammation in cardiac valves. Circulation 2001; 103(11): 1522-8.

[49] Freeman RV, Otto CM. Spectrum of calcific aortic valve disease: pathogenesis, disease progression, and treatment strategies. Circulation 2005; 111(24): 3316-26.

[50] Chan KL, Ghani M, Woodend K, Burwash IG. Case-controlled study to assess risk factors for aortic stenosis in congenitally bicuspid aortic valve. Am J Cardiol 2001; 88(6): 690-3.

[51] Mautner GC, Mautner SL, Cannon RO, 3rd, Hunsberger SA, Roberts WC. Clinical factors useful in predicting aortic valve structure in patients > 40 years of age with isolated valvular aortic stenosis. Am J Cardiol 1993; 72(2): 194-8.

[52] Robinson PN, Godfrey M. The molecular genetics of Marfan syndrome and related microfibrillopathies. J Med Genet 2000; 37(1): 9-25.

[53] Guntheroth WG. A critical review of the American College of Cardiology/American Heart Association practice guidelines on bicuspid aortic valve with dilated ascending aorta. Am J Cardiol 2008; 102(1): 107-10.

[54] Holman E. The obscure physiology of poststenotic dilatation; its relation to the development of aneurysms. J Thorac Surg 1954; 28(2): 109-33.

[55] Guntheroth WG. Causes and effects of poststenotic dilation of the pulmonary trunk. Am J Cardiol 2002; 89(6): 774-6.

[56] Bruns DL, Connolly JE, Holman E, Stofer RC. Experimental observations on post-stenotic dilatation. J Thorac Cardiovasc Surg 1959; 38: 662-9.

[57] McCrindle BW. Independent predictors of immediate results of percutaneous balloon aortic valvotomy in children. Valvuloplasty and Angioplasty of Congenital Anomalies (VACA) Registry Investigators. Am J Cardiol 1996; 77(4): 286-93.

[58] Kouchoukos NT, Davila-Roman VG, Spray TL, Murphy SF, Perrillo JB. Replacement of the aortic root with a pulmonary autograft in children and young adults with aortic-valve disease. N Engl J Med 1994; 330(1): 1-6.

[59] Ross DN. Replacement of aortic and mitral valves with a pulmonary autograft. Lancet 1967; 2(7523): 956-8.

[60] Raja SG, Pollock JC. Current outcomes of Ross operation for pediatric and adolescent patients. J Heart Valve Dis 2007; 16(1): 27-36.

[61] Selzer A. Changing aspects of the natural history of valvular aortic stenosis. N Engl J Med 1987; 317(2): 91-8.

[62] Dare AJ, Veinot JP, Edwards WD, Tazelaar HD, Schaff HV. New observations on the etiology of aortic valve disease: a surgical pathologic study of 236 cases from 1990. Hum Pathol 1993; 24(12): 1330-8.

[63] Stephan PJ, Henry AC, 3rd, Hebeler RF, Jr., Whiddon L, Roberts WC. Comparison of age, gender, number of aortic valve cusps, concomitant coronary artery bypass grafting, and magnitude of left ventricular-systemic arterial peak systolic gradient in adults having aortic valve replacement for isolated aortic valve stenosis. Am J Cardiol 1997; 79(2): 166-72.

[64] Lindroos M, Kupari M, Heikkila J, Tilvis R. Prevalence of aortic valve abnormalities in the elderly: an echocardiographic study of a random population sample. J Am Coll Cardiol 1993; 21(5): 1220-5.

[65] O'Keefe JH, Jr., Vlietstra RE, Bailey KR, Holmes DR, Jr. Natural history of candidates for balloon aortic valvuloplasty. Mayo Clin Proc 1987; 62(11): 986-91.

[66] Otto CM, Kuusisto J, Reichenbach DD, Gown AM, O'Brien KD. Characterization of the early lesion of 'degenerative' valvular aortic stenosis. Histological and immunohistochemical studies. Circulation 1994; 90(2): 844-53.

[67] O'Brien KD, Reichenbach DD, Marcovina SM, Kuusisto J, Alpers CE, Otto CM. Apolipoproteins B, (a), and E accumulate in the morphologically early lesion of 'degenerative' valvular aortic stenosis. Arterioscler Thromb Vasc Biol 1996; 16(4): 523-32.

[68] Olsson M, Thyberg J, Nilsson J. Presence of oxidized low density lipoprotein in nonrheumatic stenotic aortic valves. Arterioscler Thromb Vasc Biol 1999; 19(5): 1218-22.

[69] Olsson M, Dalsgaard CJ, Haegerstrand A, Rosenqvist M, Ryden L, Nilsson J. Accumulation of T lymphocytes and expression of interleukin-2 receptors in nonrheumatic stenotic aortic valves. J Am Coll Cardiol 1994; 23(5): 1162-70.

[70] Wallby L, Janerot-Sjoberg B, Steffensen T, Broqvist M. T lymphocyte infiltration in non-rheumatic aortic stenosis: a comparative descriptive study between tricuspid and bicuspid aortic valves. Heart 2002; 88(4): 348-51.

[71] Ghaisas NK, Foley JB, O'Briain DS, Crean P, Kelleher D, Walsh M. Adhesion molecules in nonrheumatic aortic valve disease: endothelial expression, serum levels and effects of valve replacement. J Am Coll Cardiol 2000; 36(7): 2257-62.

[72] Kaden JJ, Dempfle CE, Grobholz R, Tran HT, Kilic R, Sarikoc A, et al. Interleukin-1 beta promotes matrix metalloproteinase expression and cell proliferation in calcific aortic valve stenosis. Atherosclerosis 2003; 170(2): 205-11.

[73] Ross R. Atherosclerosis is an inflammatory disease. Am Heart J 1999; 138(5 Pt 2): S419-20.

[74] Thompson JB, Blaha M, Resar JR, Blumenthal RS, Desai MY. Strategies to reverse atherosclerosis: an imaging perspective. Curr Treat Options Cardiovasc Med 2008; 10(4): 283-93.

[75] Nicholls SJ, Tuzcu EM, Sipahi I, Grasso AW, Schoenhagen P, Hu T, et al. Statins, high-density lipoprotein cholesterol, and regression of coronary atherosclerosis. Jama 2007; 297(5): 499-508.

[76] Watanabe K, Sugiyama S, Kugiyama K, Honda O, Fukushima H, Koga H, et al. Stabilization of carotid atheroma assessed by quantitative ultrasound analysis in nonhypercholesterolemic patients with coronary artery disease. J Am Coll Cardiol 2005; 46(11): 2022-30.

[77] Moura LM, Ramos SF, Zamorano JL, Barros IM, Azevedo LF, Rocha-Goncalves F, et al. Rosuvastatin affecting aortic valve endothelium to slow the progression of aortic stenosis. J Am Coll Cardiol 2007; 49(5): 554-61.

[78] Cowell SJ, Newby DE, Prescott RJ, Bloomfield P, Reid J, Northridge DB, et al. A randomized trial of intensive lipid-lowering therapy in calcific aortic stenosis. N Engl J Med 2005; 352(23): 2389-97.

[79] Rossebo AB, Pedersen TR, Boman K, Brudi P, Chambers JB, Egstrup K, et al. Intensive lipid lowering with simvastatin and ezetimibe in aortic stenosis. N Engl J Med 2008; 359(13): 1343-56.

[80] Schwarz F, Baumann P, Manthey J, Hoffmann M, Schuler G, Mehmel HC, et al. The effect of aortic valve replacement on survival. Circulation 1982; 66(5): 1105-10.

[81] Ross J, Jr., Braunwald E. Aortic stenosis. Circulation 1968; 38(1 Suppl): 61-7.

[82] Turina J, Hess O, Sepulcri F, Krayenbuehl HP. Spontaneous course of aortic valve disease. Eur Heart J 1987; 8(5): 471-83.

[83] Horstkotte D, Loogen F. The natural history of aortic valve stenosis. Eur Heart J 1988; 9 Suppl E: 57-64.

[84] Levinson JR, Akins CW, Buckley MJ, Newell JB, Palacios IF, Block PC, et al. Octogenarians with aortic stenosis. Outcome after aortic valve replacement. Circulation 1989; 80(3 Pt 1): I49-56.

[85] Iung B, Cachier A, Baron G, Messika-Zeitoun D, Delahaye F, Tornos P, et al. Decision-making in elderly patients with severe aortic stenosis: why are so many denied surgery? Eur Heart J 2005; 26(24): 2714-20.

[86] Bouma BJ, van der Meulen JH, van den Brink RB, Arnold AE, Smidts A, Teunter LH, et al. Variability in treatment advice for elderly patients with aortic stenosis: a nationwide survey in The Netherlands. Heart 2001; 85(2): 196-201.

[87] Charlson E, Legedza AT, Hamel MB. Decision-making and outcomes in severe symptomatic aortic stenosis. J Heart Valve Dis 2006; 15(3): 312-21.

[88] Bach DS, Cimino N, Deeb GM. Unoperated patients with severe aortic stenosis. J Am Coll Cardiol 2007; 50(20): 2018-9.

[89] Webb JG, Pasupati S, Humphries K, Thompson C, Altwegg L, Moss R, et al. Percutaneous transarterial aortic valve replacement in selected high-risk patients with aortic stenosis. Circulation 2007; 116(7): 755-63.

[90]   Cribier A, Eltchaninoff H, Bash A, Borenstein N, Tron C, Bauer F, *et al.* Percutaneous transcatheter implantation of an aortic valve prosthesis for calcific aortic stenosis: first human case description. Circulation 2002; 106(24): 3006-8.

[91]   Cribier A, Eltchaninoff H, Tron C, Bauer F, Agatiello C, Sebagh L, *et al.* Early experience with percutaneous transcatheter implantation of heart valve prosthesis for the treatment of end-stage inoperable patients with calcific aortic stenosis. J Am Coll Cardiol 2004; 43(4): 698-703.

[92]   Webb JG, Chandavimol M, Thompson CR, Ricci DR, Carere RG, Munt BI, *et al.* Percutaneous aortic valve implantation retrograde from the femoral artery. Circulation 2006; 113(6): 842-50.

[93]   Lichtenstein SV, Cheung A, Ye J, Thompson CR, Carere RG, Pasupati S, *et al.* Transapical transcatheter aortic valve implantation in humans: initial clinical experience. Circulation 2006; 114(6): 591-6.

[94]   Grube E, Laborde JC, Zickmann B, Gerckens U, Felderhoff T, Sauren B, *et al.* First report on a human percutaneous transluminal implantation of a self-expanding valve prosthesis for interventional treatment of aortic valve stenosis. Catheter Cardiovasc Interv 2005; 66(4): 465-9.

[95]   Grube E, Laborde JC, Gerckens U, Felderhoff T, Sauren B, Buellesfeld L, *et al.* Percutaneous implantation of the CoreValve self-expanding valve prosthesis in high-risk patients with aortic valve disease: the Siegburg first-in-man study. Circulation 2006; 114(15): 1616-24.

[96]   McKay RG, Safian RD, Lock JE, Mandell VS, Thurer RL, Schnitt SJ, *et al.* Balloon dilatation of calcific aortic stenosis in elderly patients: postmortem, intraoperative, and percutaneous valvuloplasty studies. Circulation 1986; 74(1): 119-25.

[97]   Safian RD, Mandell VS, Thurer RE, Hutchins GM, Schnitt SJ, Grossman W, *et al.* Postmortem and intraoperative balloon valvuloplasty of calcific aortic stenosis in elderly patients: mechanisms of successful dilation. J Am Coll Cardiol 1987; 9(3): 655-60.

[98]   Isner JM, Samuels DA, Slovenkai GA, Halaburka KR, Hougen TJ, Desnoyers MR, *et al.* Mechanism of aortic balloon valvuloplasty: fracture of valvular calcific deposits. Ann Intern Med 1988; 108(3): 377-80.

[99]   Block PC, Palacios IF. Clinical and hemodynamic follow-up after percutaneous aortic valvuloplasty in the elderly. Am J Cardiol 1988; 62(10 Pt 1): 760-3.

[100]   Ferguson JJ, 3rd, Riuli EP, Massumi A, Treistman B, Edelman SK, Harlan MV, *et al.* Balloon aortic valvuloplasty: the Texas Heart Institute experience. Tex Heart Inst J 1990; 17(1): 23-30.

[101]   Berland J, Cribier A, Savin T, Lefebvre E, Koning R, Letac B. Percutaneous balloon valvuloplasty in patients with severe aortic stenosis and low ejection fraction. Immediate results and 1-year follow-up. Circulation 1989; 79(6): 1189-96.

[102]   Davidson CJ, Harrison JK, Leithe ME, Kisslo KB, Bashore TM. Failure of balloon aortic valvuloplasty to result in sustained clinical improvement in patients with depressed left ventricular function. Am J Cardiol 1990; 65(1): 72-7.

[103]   Otto CM, Mickel MC, Kennedy JW, Alderman EL, Bashore TM, Block PC, *et al.* Three-year outcome after balloon aortic valvuloplasty. Insights into prognosis of valvular aortic stenosis. Circulation 1994; 89(2): 642-50.

[104]   Lieberman EB, Bashore TM, Hermiller JB, Wilson JS, Pieper KS, Keeler GP, *et al.* Balloon aortic valvuloplasty in adults: failure of procedure to improve long-term survival. J Am Coll Cardiol 1995; 26(6): 1522-8.

[105]   Kuntz RE, Tosteson AN, Berman AD, Goldman L, Gordon PC, Leonard BM, *et al.* Predictors of event-free survival after balloon aortic valvuloplasty. N Engl J Med 1991; 325(1): 17-23.

[106]   Brady ST, Davis CA, Kussmaul WG, Laskey WK, Hirshfeld JW, Jr., Herrmann HC. Percutaneous aortic balloon valvuloplasty in octogenarians: morbidity and mortality. Ann Intern Med 1989; 110(10): 761-6.

[107]   Letac B, Cribier A, Koning R, Bellefleur JP. Results of percutaneous transluminal valvuloplasty in 218 adults with valvular aortic stenosis. Am J Cardiol 1988; 62(9): 598-605.

[108]   Sherman W, Hershman R, Lazzam C, Cohen M, Ambrose J, Gorlin R. Balloon valvuloplasty in adult aortic stenosis: determinants of clinical outcome. Ann Intern Med 1989; 110(6): 421-5.

[109]   Zipes L, Bonow, Braunwald. Braunwald's Heart Disease. 7th ed; 2005.

[110]   Hanson TP, Edwards BS, Edwards JE. Pathology of surgically excised mitral valves. One hundred consecutive cases. Arch Pathol Lab Med 1985; 109(9): 823-8.

[111]   Olsen LJ, Subramanian R, Ackermann DM, Edwards WD. Surgical pathology of the mitral valve: a study of 712 cases spanning 21 years. Mayo Clinic Proc 1987; 62: 22-34.

[112]   Padmavati S. Rheumatic fever and rheumatic heart disease in India at the turn of the century. Indian Heart J 2001; 53(1): 35-7.

[113]   Horstkotte D, Niehues R, Strauer BE. Pathomorphological aspects, aetiology and natural history of acquired mitral valve stenosis. Eur Heart J 1991; 12 Suppl B: 55-60.

[114]   Iung B, Baron G, Butchart EG, Delahaye F, Gohlke-Barwolf C, Levang OW, *et al.* A prospective survey of patients with valvular heart disease in Europe: The Euro Heart Survey on Valvular Heart Disease. Eur Heart J 2003; 24(13): 1231-43.

[115]   Carroll JD, Feldman T. Percutaneous mitral balloon valvotomy and the new demographics of mitral stenosis. Jama 1993; 270(14): 1731-6.

[116] Carpentier AF, Pellerin M, Fuzellier JF, Relland JY. Extensive calcification of the mitral valve anulus: pathology and surgical management. J Thorac Cardiovasc Surg 1996; 111(4): 718-29; discussion 729-30.

[117] Hammer WJ, Roberts WC, deLeon AC. "Mitral stenosis" secondary to combined "massive" mitral anular calcific deposits and small, hypertrophied left ventricles. Hemodynamic documentation in four patients. Am J Med 1978; 64(3): 371-6.

[118] Akram MR, Chan T, McAuliffe S, Chenzbraun A. Non-rheumatic annular mitral stenosis: prevalence and characteristics. Eur J Echocardiogr 2009; 10(1): 103-5.

[119] Davachi F, Moller JH, Edwards JE. Diseases of the mitral valve in infancy. An anatomic analysis of 55 cases. Circulation 1971; 43(4): 565-79.

[120] Ruckman RN, Van Praagh R. Anatomic types of congenital mitral stenosis: report of 49 autopsy cases with consideration of diagnosis and surgical implications. Am J Cardiol 1978; 42(4): 592-601.

[121] Pellikka PA, Tajik AJ, Khandheria BK, Seward JB, Callahan JA, Pitot HC, *et al.* Carcinoid heart disease. Clinical and echocardiographic spectrum in 74 patients. Circulation 1993; 87(4): 1188-96.

[122] Leder AA, Bosworth WC. Angiokeratoma Corporis Diffusum Universale (Fabry's Disease) With Mitral Stenosis. Am J Med 1965; 38: 814-9.

[123] Waller BF, McManus BM, Roberts WC. Mitral valve stenosis produced by or worsened by active bacterial endocarditis. Chest 1982; 82(4): 498-500.

[124] Roberts WC, Virmani R. Aschoff bodies at necropsy in valvular heart disease. Evidence from an analysis of 543 patients over 14 years of age that rheumatic heart disease, at least anatomically, is a disease of the mitral valve. Circulation 1978; 57(4): 803-7.

[125] Golbasi Z, Ucar O, Keles T, Sahin A, Cagli K, Camsari A, *et al.* Increased levels of high sensitive C-reactive protein in patients with chronic rheumatic valve disease: evidence of ongoing inflammation. Eur J Heart Fail 2002; 4(5): 593-5.

[126] Ellis NM, Li Y, Hildebrand W, Fischetti VA, Cunningham MW. T cell mimicry and epitope specificity of cross-reactive T cell clones from rheumatic heart disease. J Immunol 2005; 175(8): 5448-56.

[127] D'Cruz IA, Cohen HC, Prabhu R, Bisla V, Glick G. Clinical manifestations of mitral annulus calcification, with emphasis on its echocardiographic features. Am Heart J 1977; 94(3): 367-77.

[128] Labovitz AJ, Nelson JG, Windhorst DM, Kennedy HL, Williams GA. Frequency of mitral valve dysfunction from mitral anular calcium as detected by Doppler echocardiography. Am J Cardiol 1985; 55(1): 133-7.

[129] Ramirez J, Flowers NC. Severe mitral stenosis secondary to massive calcification of the mitral annulus with unusual echocardiographic manifestations. Clin Cardiol 1980; 3(4): 284-7.

[130] Osterberger LE, Goldstein S, Khaja F, Lakier JB. Functional mitral stenosis in patients with massive mitral annular calcification. Circulation 1981; 64(3): 472-6.

[131] Muddassir SM, Pressman GS. Mitral annular calcification as a cause of mitral valve gradients. Int J Cardiol 2007; 123(1): 58-62.

[132] Rowe JC, Bland EF, Sprague HB, White PD. The course of mitral stenosis without surgery: ten- and twenty-year perspectives. Ann Intern Med 1960; 52: 741-9.

[133] Olesen KH. The natural history of 271 patients with mitral stenosis under medical treatment. Br Heart J 1962; 24: 349-57.

[134] Vijaykumar M, Narula J, Reddy KS. Incidence of rheumatic fever and prevelence of rheumatic heart disease in India. Int J Cardiol 1992; 43: 221-228.

[135] Joswig BC, Glover MU, Handler JB, Warren SE, Vieweg WV. Contrasting progression of mitral stenosis in Malayans versus American-born Caucasians. Am Heart J 1982; 104(6): 1400-3.

[136] Selzer A, Cohn KE. Natural history of mitral stenosis: a review. Circulation 1972; 45(4): 878-90.

[137] Marzo KP, Herling IM. Valvular disease in the elderly. Cardiovasc Clin 1993; 23: 175-207.

[138] Fox CS, Vasan RS, Parise H, Levy D, O'Donnell CJ, D'Agostino RB, *et al.* Mitral annular calcification predicts cardiovascular morbidity and mortality: the Framingham Heart Study. Circulation 2003; 107(11): 1492-6.

[139] Tenenbaum A, Shemesh J, Fisman EZ, Motro M. Advanced mitral annular calcification is associated with severe coronary calcification on fast dual spiral computed tomography. Invest Radiol 2000; 35(3): 193-8.

[140] Hugenholtz PG, Ryan TJ, Stein SW, Abelmann WH. The spectrum of pure mitral stenosis. Hemodynamic studies in relation to clinical disability. Am J Cardiol 1962; 10: 773-84.

[141] Kasalicky J, Hurych J, Widimsky J, Dejdar R, Metys R, Stanek V. Left heart haemodynamics at rest and during exercise in patients with mitral stenosis. Br Heart J 1968; 30(2): 188-95.

[142] Braunwald E, Moscovitz HL, Amram SS, Lasser RP, Sapin SO, Himmelstein A, *et al.* The hemodynamics of the left side of the heart as studied by simultaneous left atrial, left ventricular, and aortic pressures; particular reference to mitral stenosis. Circulation 1955; 12(1): 69-81.

[143] Tamai J, Yoshioka T, Yasuda S, Takaki H, Okano Y, Ishikura F, *et al.* Increase in peak oxygen uptake by restoration of atrial contraction in patients after percutaneous transvenous mitral commissurotomy. J Heart Valve Dis 1993; 2(6): 623-8.

[144] Vora A, Karnad D, Goyal V, Naik A, Gupta A, Lokhandwala Y, *et al.* Control of rate versus rhythm in rheumatic atrial fibrillation: a randomized study. Indian Heart J 2004; 56(2): 110-6.

[145] Otto CM, Davis KB, Reid CL, Slater JN, Kronzon I, Kisslo KB, *et al.* Relation between pulmonary artery pressure and mitral stenosis severity in patients undergoing balloon mitral commissurotomy. Am J Cardiol 1993; 71(10): 874-8.

[146] Ward C, Hancock BW. Extreme pulmonary hypertension caused by mitral valve disease. Natural history and results of surgery. Br Heart J 1975; 37(1): 74-8.

[147] Levine MJ, Weinstein JS, Diver DJ, Berman AD, Wyman RM, Cunningham MJ, *et al.* Progressive improvement in pulmonary vascular resistance after percutaneous mitral valvuloplasty. Circulation 1989; 79(5): 1061-7.

[148] Georgeson S, Panidis IP, Kleaveland JP, Heilbrunn S, Gonzales R. Effect of percutaneous balloon valvuloplasty on pulmonary hypertension in mitral stenosis. Am Heart J 1993; 125(5 Pt 1): 1374-9.

[149] Palacios IF, Sanchez PL, Harrell LC, Weyman AE, Block PC. Which patients benefit from percutaneous mitral balloon valvuloplasty? Prevalvuloplasty and postvalvuloplasty variables that predict long-term outcome. Circulation 2002; 105(12): 1465-71.

[150] Cutler EC, Levine SA. Cardiotomy and valvulotomy for mitral stenosis: experimental observations and clinical notes concerning an operated case with recovery. Bost Med Surg J 1923; 188: 1023-7.

[151] Suttar HS. The surgical treatment of mitral stenosis. BMJ 1925; 2: 603-6.

[152] Bailey CP. The surgical treatment of mitral stenosis (mitral commissurotomy). Dis Chest 1949; 15(4): 377-97.

[153] Harken DE, Ellis LB, *et al.* The surgical treatment of mitral stenosis; valvuloplasty. N Engl J Med 1948; 239(22): 801-9.

[154] Inoue K, Owaki T, Nakamura T, Kitamura F, Miyamoto N. Clinical application of transvenous mitral commissurotomy by a new balloon catheter. J Thorac Cardiovasc Surg 1984; 87(3): 394-402.

[155] Kaplan JD, Isner JM, Karas RH, Halaburka KR, Konstam MA, Hougen TJ, *et al. In vitro* analysis of mechanisms of balloon valvuloplasty of stenotic mitral valves. Am J Cardiol 1987; 59(4): 318-23.

[156] McKay RG, Lock JE, Safian RD, Come PC, Diver DJ, Baim DS, *et al.* Balloon dilation of mitral stenosis in adult patients: postmortem and percutaneous mitral valvuloplasty studies. J Am Coll Cardiol 1987; 9(4): 723-31.

[157] Wilkins GT, Weyman AE, Abascal VM, Block PC, Palacios IF. Percutaneous balloon dilatation of the mitral valve: an analysis of echocardiographic variables related to outcome and the mechanism of dilatation. Br Heart J 1988; 60(4): 299-308.

[158] Fatkin D, Roy P, Morgan JJ, Feneley MP. Percutaneous balloon mitral valvotomy with the Inoue single-balloon catheter: commissural morphology as a determinant of outcome. J Am Coll Cardiol 1993; 21(2): 390-7.

[159] Sutaria N, Northridge DB, Shaw TR. Significance of commissural calcification on outcome of mitral balloon valvotomy. Heart 2000; 84(4): 398-402.

[160] Kronzon I, Tunick PA, Glassman E, Slater J, Schwinger M, Freedberg RS. Transesophageal echocardiography to detect atrial clots in candidates for percutaneous transseptal mitral balloon valvuloplasty. J Am Coll Cardiol 1990; 16(5): 1320-2.

[161] Nobuyoshi M, Arita T, Shirai S, Hamasaki N, Yokoi H, Iwabuchi M, *et al.* Percutaneous balloon mitral valvuloplasty: a review. Circulation 2009; 119(8): e211-9.

[162] Chen WJ, Chen MF, Liau CS, Wu CC, Lee YT. Safety of percutaneous transvenous balloon mitral commissurotomy in patients with mitral stenosis and thrombus in the left atrial appendage. Am J Cardiol 1992; 70(1): 117-9.

[163] Zhang HP, Gamra H, Allen JW, Lau FY, Ruiz CE. Balloon valvotomy for mitral stenosis associated with moderate mitral regurgitation. Am J Cardiol 1995; 75(14): 960-3.

[164] Zhang HP, Yen GS, Allen JW, Lau FY, Ruiz CE. Comparison of late results of balloon valvotomy in mitral stenosis with versus without mitral regurgitation. Am J Cardiol 1998; 81(1): 51-5.

[165] Herrmann HC, Lima JA, Feldman T, Chisholm R, Isner J, O'Neill W, *et al.* Mechanisms and outcome of severe mitral regurgitation after Inoue balloon valvuloplasty. North American Inoue Balloon Investigators. J Am Coll Cardiol 1993; 22(3): 783-9.

[166] Miche E, Fassbender D, Minami K, Gleichmann U, Mannebach H, Schmidt H, *et al.* Pathomorphological characteristics of resected mitral valves after unsuccessful valvuloplasty. J Cardiovasc Surg (Torino) 1996; 37(5): 475-81.

[167] Inoue K, Kitamura F, Chikusa H, Miyamoto N. Atrial septostomy by a new balloon catheter. Jpn Circ J 1981; 45: 730-8.

[168] Inoue K, Nakamura T, Kitamura F. Nonoperative mitral commissurotomy by a new balloon catheter. Jpn Circ J 1982; 46: 877.

[169] Inoue K. Percutaneous transvenous mitral commissurotomy using the Inoue balloon. Eur Heart J 1991; 12 Suppl B: 99-108.

[170] Stefanadis C, Stratos C, Pitsavos C, Kallikazaros I, Triposkiadis F, Trikas A, *et al.* Retrograde nontransseptal balloon mitral valvuloplasty. Immediate results and long-term follow-up. Circulation 1992; 85(5): 1760-7.

[171] Thomas JD, Wilkins GT, Choong CY, Abascal VM, Palacios IF, Block PC, *et al.* Inaccuracy of mitral pressure half-time immediately after percutaneous mitral valvotomy. Dependence on transmitral gradient and left atrial and ventricular compliance. Circulation 1988; 78(4): 980-93.

[172] Cormier B, Vahanian A, Michel PL, Porte JM, Iung B, Dadez E, *et al.* Transoesophageal echocardiography in the assessment of percutaneous mitral commissurotomy. Eur Heart J 1991; 12 Suppl B: 61-5.

[173] Cequier A, Bonan R, Serra A, Dyrda I, Crepeau J, Dethy M, *et al.* Left-to-right atrial shunting after percutaneous mitral valvuloplasty. Incidence and long-term hemodynamic follow-up. Circulation 1990; 81(4): 1190-7.

[174] Yoshida K, Yoshikawa J, Akasaka T, Yamaura Y, Shakudo M, Hozumi T, *et al.* Assessment of left-to-right atrial shunting after percutaneous mitral valvuloplasty by transesophageal color Doppler flow-mapping. Circulation 1989; 80(6): 1521-6.

[175] Hernandez R, Banuelos C, Alfonso F, Goicolea J, Fernandez-Ortiz A, Escaned J, et al. Long-term clinical and echocardiographic follow-up after percutaneous mitral valvuloplasty with the Inoue balloon. Circulation 1999; 99(12): 1580-6.

[176] Chen CR, Cheng TO. Percutaneous balloon mitral valvuloplasty by the Inoue technique: a multicenter study of 4832 patients in China. Am Heart J 1995; 129(6): 1197-203.

[177] Neumayer U, Schmidt HK, Fassbender D, Mannebach H, Bogunovic N, Horstkotte D. Early (three-month) results of percutaneous mitral valvotomy with the Inoue balloon in 1,123 consecutive patients comparing various age groups. Am J Cardiol 2002; 90(2): 190-3.

[178] Iung B, Nicoud-Houel A, Fondard O, Hafid A, Haghighat T, Brochet E, *et al.* Temporal trends in percutaneous mitral commissurotomy over a 15-year period. Eur Heart J 2004; 25(8): 701-7.

[179] Reyes VP, Raju BS, Wynne J, Stephenson LW, Raju R, Fromm BS, *et al.* Percutaneous balloon valvuloplasty compared with open surgical commissurotomy for mitral stenosis. N Engl J Med 1994; 331(15): 961-7.

[180] Ben Farhat M, Ayari M, Maatouk F, Betbout F, Gamra H, Jarra M, *et al.* Percutaneous balloon versus surgical closed and open mitral commissurotomy: seven-year follow-up results of a randomized trial. Circulation 1998; 97(3): 245-50.

[181] Tanabe Y, Oshima M, Suzuki M, Takahashi M. Determinants of delayed improvement in exercise capacity after percutaneous transvenous mitral commissurotomy. Am Heart J 2000; 139(5): 889-94.

[182] Krishnamoorthy KM, Dash PK, Radhakrishnan S, Shrivastava S. Response of different grades of pulmonary artery hypertension to balloon mitral valvuloplasty. Am J Cardiol 2002; 90(10): 1170-3.

[183] Iung B, Garbarz E, Michaud P, Helou S, Farah B, Berdah P, *et al.* Late results of percutaneous mitral commissurotomy in a series of 1024 patients. Analysis of late clinical deterioration: frequency, anatomic findings, and predictive factors. Circulation 1999; 99(25): 3272-8.

[184] Lock JE, Khalilullah M, Shrivastava S, Bahl V, Keane JF. Percutaneous catheter commissurotomy in rheumatic mitral stenosis. N Engl J Med 1985; 313(24): 1515-8.

[185] Al Zaibag M, Ribeiro PA, Al Kasab S, Al Fagih MR. Percutaneous double-balloon mitral valvotomy for rheumatic mitral-valve stenosis. Lancet 1986; 1(8484): 757-61.

[186] Bonhoeffer P, Esteves C, Casal U, Tortoledo F, Yonga G, Patel T, *et al.* Percutaneous mitral valve dilatation with the Multi-Track System. Catheter Cardiovasc Interv 1999; 48(2): 178-83.

[187] Park SJ, Kim JJ, Park SW, Song JK, Doo YC, Lee SJ. Immediate and one-year results of percutaneous mitral balloon valvuloplasty using Inoue and double-balloon techniques. Am J Cardiol 1993; 71(11): 938-43.

[188] Trevino AJ, Ibarra M, Garcia A, Uribe A, de la Fuente F, Bonfil MA, *et al.* Immediate and long-term results of balloon mitral commissurotomy for rheumatic mitral stenosis: comparison between Inoue and double-balloon techniques. Am Heart J 1996; 131(3): 530-6.

[189] Bassand JP, Schiele F, Bernard Y, Anguenot T, Payet M, Ba SA, *et al.* The double-balloon and Inoue techniques in percutaneous mitral valvuloplasty: comparative results in a series of 232 cases. J Am Coll Cardiol 1991; 18(4): 982-9.

[190] Cribier A, Eltchaninoff H, Koning R, Rath PC, Arora R, Imam A, *et al.* Percutaneous mechanical mitral commissurotomy with a newly designed metallic valvulotome: immediate results of the initial experience in 153 patients. Circulation 1999; 99(6): 793-9.

[191] Chen GY, Tseng CD, Chiang FT, Hsu KL, Lo HM, Tseng YZ, *et al.* Congenital mitral stenosis: challenge of percutaneous transvenous mitral commissurotomy. Int J Cardiol 1997; 60(1): 99-102.

[192] de Souza JA, Martinez EE, Jr., Ambrose JA, Alves CM, Born D, Buffolo E, *et al.* Percutaneous balloon mitral valvuloplasty in comparison with open mitral valve commissurotomy for mitral stenosis during pregnancy. J Am Coll Cardiol 2001; 37(3): 900-3.

[193] Ribeiro PA, Fawzy ME, Awad M, Dunn B, Duran CG. Balloon valvotomy for pregnant patients with severe pliable mitral stenosis using the Inoue technique with total abdominal and pelvic shielding. Am Heart J 1992; 124(6): 1558-62.

[194] Kultursay H, Turkoglu C, Akin M, Payzin S, Soydas C, Akilli A. Mitral balloon valvuloplasty with transesophageal echocardiography without using fluoroscopy. Cathet Cardiovasc Diagn 1992; 27(4): 317-21.

[195] hTuzcu EM, Block PC, Griffin BP, Newell JB, Palacios IF. Immediate and long-term outcome of percutaneous mitral valvotomy in patients 65 years and older. Circulation 1992; 85(3): 963-71.

[196] Hildick-Smith DJ, Taylor GJ, Shapiro LM. Inoue balloon mitral valvuloplasty: long-term clinical and echocardiographic follow-up of a predominantly unfavourable population. Eur Heart J 2000; 21(20): 1690-7.

[197] Otto CM. Valvular Heart Disease pp 415-436. 2nd ed: Philadelphia, WB Saunders; 2004.

[198] Rao PS. Transcatheter treatment of pulmonary outflow tract obstruction: a review. Prog Cardiovasc Dis 1992; 35(2): 119-58.

[199] Jackson MW, KP; Peart I *et al.* Epidemiology of congenital heart disease in Merseyside 1978-1988. Cardiol Young 1996(6): 272-80.

[200] Nugent EW, Freedom RM, Nora JJ, Ellison RC, Rowe RD, Nadas AS. Clinical course in pulmonary stenosis. Circulation 1977; 56(1 Suppl): I38-47.

[201] Mody MR. The natural history of uncomplicated valvular pulmonic stenosis. Am Heart J 1975; 90(3): 317-21.

[202] Marantz PM, Huhta JC, Mullins CE, Murphy DJ, Jr., Nihill MR, Ludomirsky A, *et al.* Results of balloon valvuloplasty in typical and dysplastic pulmonary valve stenosis: Doppler echocardiographic follow-up. J Am Coll Cardiol 1988; 12(2): 476-9.

[203] Rao PS. Balloon pulmonary valvuloplasty: a review. Clin Cardiol 1989; 12(2): 55-74.

[204] Rubio V LLR. Treatment of pulmonary valvular stenosis and tricuspid stenosis using a modified catheter. Second World Congress on Cardiology, Washington DC, 1956. Program Abstracts II,205. 1956.

[205] Semb BK, Tjonneland S, Stake G, Aabyholm G. "Balloon valvulotomy" of congenital pulmonary valve stenosis with tricuspid valve insufficiency. Cardiovasc Radiol 1979; 2(4): 239-41.

[206] Kan JS, White RI, Jr., Mitchell SE, Gardner TJ. Percutaneous balloon valvuloplasty: a new method for treating congenital pulmonary-valve stenosis. N Engl J Med 1982; 307(9): 540-2.

[207] Rao PS. Percutaneous balloon pulmonary valvuloplasty: state of the art. Catheter Cardiovasc Interv 2007; 69(5): 747-63.

[208] Musewe NN, Robertson MA, Benson LN, Smallhorn JF, Burrows PE, Freedom RM, *et al.* The dysplastic pulmonary valve: echocardiographic features and results of balloon dilatation. Br Heart J 1987; 57(4): 364-70.

[209] DiSessa TG, Alpert BS, Chase NA, Birnbaum SE, Watson DC. Balloon valvuloplasty in children with dysplastic pulmonary valves. Am J Cardiol 1987; 60(4): 405-7.

[210] Rey C, Marache P, Francart C, Dupuis C. Percutaneous transluminal balloon valvuloplasty of congenital pulmonary valve stenosis, with a special report on infants and neonates. J Am Coll Cardiol 1988; 11(4): 815-20.

[211] Radtke W, Keane JF, Fellows KE, Lang P, Lock JE. Percutaneous balloon valvotomy of congenital pulmonary stenosis using oversized balloons. J Am Coll Cardiol 1986; 8(4): 909-15.

[212] Rao PS. Further observations on the effect of balloon size on the short term and intermediate term results of balloon dilatation of the pulmonary valve. Br Heart J 1988; 60(6): 507-11.

[213] McCrindle BW. Independent predictors of long-term results after balloon pulmonary valvuloplasty. Valvuloplasty and Angioplasty of Congenital Anomalies (VACA) Registry Investigators. Circulation 1994; 89(4): 1751-9.

[214] Stanger P, Cassidy SC, Girod DA, Kan JS, Lababidi Z, Shapiro SR. Balloon pulmonary valvuloplasty: results of the Valvuloplasty and Angioplasty of Congenital Anomalies Registry. Am J Cardiol 1990; 65(11): 775-83.

[215] Thapar MK, Rao PS. Use of propranolol for severe dynamic infundibular obstruction prior to balloon pulmonary valvuloplasty (a brief communication). Cathet Cardiovasc Diagn 1990; 19(4): 240-1.

[216] Fawzy ME, Hassan W, Fadel BM, Sergani H, El Shaer F, El Widaa H, *et al.* Long-term results (up to 17 years) of pulmonary balloon valvuloplasty in adults and its effects on concomitant severe infundibular stenosis and tricuspid regurgitation. Am Heart J 2007; 153(3): 433-8.

[217] Kaul UA, Singh B, Tyagi S, Bhargava M, Arora R, Khalilullah M. Long-term results after balloon pulmonary valvuloplasty in adults. Am Heart J 1993; 126(5): 1152-5.

[218] Rao PS, Galal O, Patnana M, Buck SH, Wilson AD. Results of three to 10 year follow up of balloon dilatation of the pulmonary valve. Heart 1998; 80(6): 591-5.

[219] Earing MG, Connolly HM, Dearani JA, Ammash NM, Grogan M, Warnes CA. Long-term follow-up of patients after surgical treatment for isolated pulmonary valve stenosis. Mayo Clin Proc 2005; 80(7): 871-6.

[220] Rao PS. Balloon pulmonary valvuloplasty for isolated pulmonic stenosis. In: Transcatheter therapy in Pediatric Cardiology. New York; 1993.

CHAPTER 5

Percutaneous Treatment of Mitral Regurgitation Using 'Leaflet' Technologies

Rebecca Schofield[*]

Peterborough and Stamford NHS Trust Hospital, Peterborough, UK

Abstract: Mitral Regurgitation presents a significant health burden to patients and the resources of the NHS. It is the most common form of cardiac valve disease affecting more than 150 million people worldwide [1]. Typically treatment has been symptom management until such time that there is evidence of adverse ventricular remodeling or a failing left ventricle. At this time surgery can be offered in the form of mitral valve repair or replacement.

The aetiology of mitral regurgitation may to some degree define it's treatment. Currently there are a proportion of patients who would be refused conventional mitral valve surgery but would benefit from a less invasive therapy.

Newer technology is facilitating a percutaneous approach to the treatment of mitral regurgitation. These less invasive procedures replicate the tradition surgical approaches. The benefits of minimally invasive therapeutics include the avoidance of a sternotomy, cardio-pulmonary bypass and in some cases, life-long anticoagulation. Patients also require a shorter hospital stay.

These procedures have the advantage of being an option for 'high-risk' patient groups who would have previously been declined surgery.

Clinical expertise is growing in this field and thus far safety and efficacy data look promising.

The results of the first randomized head to head trial comparing surgery with percutaeous devices are due in 2010. The outcome of this trial will have exciting implications for the field of mitral valve therapies.

ANATOMY OF THE MITRAL VALVE

The mitral valve is the left sided atrio-ventricular valve. It consists of posterior and anterior leaflets, set into an annular ring, attached to papillary muscle *via* chordae tendineae. The mitral valve opens as the left ventricle relaxes during diastole thus allowing unobstructed filling of the left ventricle. During systole the pressure within the left ventricle increases and the mitral valve closes. The papillary muscles contract with the left ventricle and increase the tension on the chordae tendinae thus preventing the leaflets from everting into the left atrium. On closure of the mitral valve, backflow of blood into the left atrium is prevented, ensuring forward flow of oxygenated blood through the aortic valve, into the aorta, and the rest of the body.

Correct functioning of the valve depends on the integrity of, and interplay between, the annulus, leaflets and subvalvular apparatus.

Annulus

The mitral annulus constitutes the anatomical junction between the ventricle and the left atrium. It is often divided into two segments, anterior and posterior, according to the site of leaflet insertion.

The anterior portion of the mitral annulus is attached to the left and right fibrous trigones and is generally more developed than the posterior annulus. The right fibrous trigone is a dense junctional area between the mitral valve, tricuspid valve, non-coronary cusp of the aortic valve annuli and the membranous septum. The left fibrous trigone is situated at the junction of both left fibrous borders of the aortic and the mitral valve annuli.

The posterior segment of the mitral valve annulus is less well developed. It is prone to increase its circumference in association with left atrial or left ventricular dilatation.

The mitral annulus is saddle shaped, and during systole the commissural areas (area where anterior and posterior leaflets come together at their insertion into the annulus) move apically while annular contraction also narrows the circumference.

*Address correspondence to Rebecca Schofield:** Peterborough and Stamford NHS Trust Hospital, Peterborough, UK; E-mail: rebeccaschofield@doctors.org

The mitral annulus is surrounded by several highly important anatomic structures, including the aortic valve, the coronary sinus, and the circumflex artery (Fig. **1**).

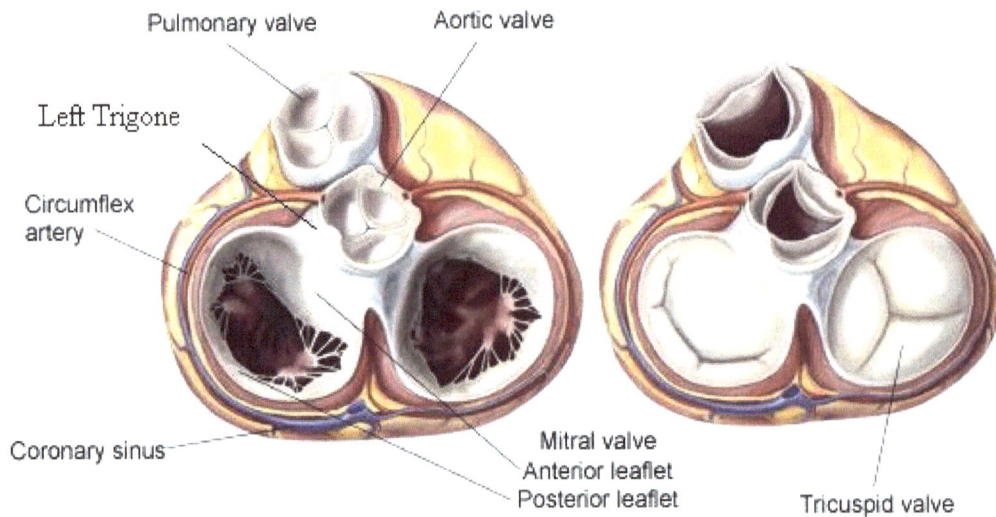

Figure 1: The Mitral Valve.

Leaflets

There are two well recognized leaflets of the mitral valve, these are named the anterior and posterior leaflets. The anterior leaflet has a semi-circular shape and attaches to one third of the annular circumference. It has considerable depth in comparison to the posterior leaflet. There is continuity between the anterior leaflet of the mitral valve and the left and non-coronary cusp of the aortic valve (the right trigone). The free edge of the anterior leaflet is usually smooth, without indentations.

The posterior leaflet of the mitral valve has a semi-lunar shape. It is attached to approximately two thirds of the annular circumference and is narrow. The posterior leaflet typically has two well defined indentations which divides the leaflet into three individual scallops identified as P1 (anterior or medial scallop), P2 (middle scallop), and P3 (posterior or lateral scallop). The three corresponding segments of the anterior leaflet are A1 (anterior segment), A2 (middle segment), and A3 (posterior segment). Indentations aid in posterior leaflet opening during diastole.

Both the anterior and posterior leaflets have similar surface areas.

Commissures

The commissures constitute a distinct area where the anterior and posterior leaflets insert into the annulus. The commissures may exist as a defined leaflet segment, but more often this area is a subtle structure.

Area of Coaptation

On the atrial surface of the anterior and posterior leaflets there are two areas. They are; the peripheral smooth area and a central rough (coaptation) area. The rough area represents the coaptation surface of the valve. The coaptation of the valve is critical to valve competency, and the depth and length of coaptation is an important assessment of mitral valve function.

Chordae Tendinae

The chordae tendinae are primarily responsible for the end-systolic position of the anterior and posterior leaflets. They arise from the papillary muscles and are classified according to their site of insertion between the free margin and the base of leaflets. Primary chordae insert on the free margin of the leaflets and function to prevent prolapse of the margin of the leaflet. Secondary chordae insert on the ventricular surface of the leaflets and relieve valvular tissue of excess tension. They may also be important in preserving ventricular shape and function. Tertiary chordae are limited to the posterior leaflet and connect the leaflet base and the mitral annulus to the papillary muscle.

Papillary Muscles and the Left Ventricle

Mitral valve function is integrally related to the left ventricle. Two papillary muscles arise from the area between the apical and middle thirds of the left ventricular wall. These are the antero-lateral papillary muscle, which often consist of one head, and the postero-medial papillary muscle with two heads. Each papillary muscle provides chordae to anterior and posterior leaflets. The antero-lateral papillary muscle blood supply is from the left anterior descending and the diagonal or a marginal branch of the circumflex artery. The blood supply to the postero-medial papillary muscle is provided by the left circumflex or right coronary artery, depending on dominance. Because of its single system of blood supply, this papillary muscle is particularly prone to injury from myocardial ischaemia. As the papillary muscles attach to the lateral wall of the left ventricle, the ventricular wall is an integral part of the mitral valve subvalvular apparatus.

PATHOPHYSIOLOGY OF MITRAL REGURGITATION

Mitral regurgitation occurs when blood flows backwards into the left atrium during systole due to a loss of integrity of the mitral valve apparatus. This may be due to dysfunction of the valve leaflets, annulus, chordae tendinae, papillary muscles, left ventricular myocardium or a combination of these.

Mitral regurgitation may be classified as degenerative or functional. Degenerative conditions cause structural pathological changes to the leaflets or the sub-valvular apparatus. Such conditions include, mitral valve prolapse and rheumatic valvular disease. Functional disease occurs in association with impaired left ventricular function, ventricular dilatation and papillary muscle dysfunction. Functional mitral regurgitation is associated with, ischaemic cardiomyopathy and non-ischaemic cardiomyopathy.

Mitral Valve Prolapse

Mitral valve prolapse (MVP) occurs when part (or all) of one (or both) of the mitral valve leaflets displace retrogradely into the left atrium during systole. The prevalence of this condition is 2-3% [2] In developed countries this is the most common cause of chronic mitral regurgitation. Several causative genetic chromosomal abnormalities have been identified however the disease may also be acquired.

Although commoner in females, more men are referred for surgery [1]. The reasons for this are unknown but may be a combination of differing natural history and referral bias.

In mitral valve prolapse, a defect in collagen results in the valve leaflets and chordae tendineae becoming baggy and fragile. As a result, on closure of the valve, the leaflets are not pulled taught and prolapse into the left atrium. The chordea are prone to rupture. These anatomical abnormalities result in inadequate coaptation. Over time annular dilatation will also occur. Hence mitral regurgitation begets mitral regurgitation.

In younger patients there may be excessive leaflet tissue, known as Barlow's syndrome [3].

The natural history of the disease is variable. Many patients may remain asymptomatic and have a near normal life-expectancy. Unfortunately, 5-10% may progress to severe mitral regurgitation [4]. Mortality amongst this group has been reported as 6.3% per annum [5]. This is comparable to the rates for triple-vessel coronary disease [6]. Common complications include; left ventricular failure, pulmonary hypertension, atrial fibrillation, endocarditis and rupture of chordae.

Patients with MVP should be closely observed and have regular assessment of the degree of mitral regurgitation, the left ventricular size and function. Patients who have symptoms or show signs of left ventricular dilatation and/or dysfunction should be considered for surgery.

The current surgical options are mitral valve replacement with a mechanical or biological prothesis or repair of the patient's native mitral valve. Mitral valve repair is becoming a more popular option with both surgeon and patient.

Although there are no randomized trials comparing mitral valve replacement and repair, a meta-analysis of observational studies favoured mitral repair in survival outcomes [7].

Repair of the native valve avoids the need for life-long anti-coagulation. The risks associated with prosthetic valves such as prosthesis failure and prosthetic-valve endocarditis are avoided. In addition in native valve repair the chordae tendinae remain intact which preserves the beneficial relationship between the subvalvular apparatus and the left ventricular wall.

The most common isolated prolapse encountered in degenerative mitral valve prolapse is that of the posterior middle scallop (P2). Repairs involving the anterior leaflet or both leaflets are more complicated. Various techniques such as triangular resection, chordal transposition, chordal shortening, artifical chordal replacement and edge-to edge repair may be used [4,8-13]. Transoesophageal echocardiography is routinely used in most centres during mitral repair procedures.

The goals of successful surgical repair are to ensure adequate surface of coaptation of both leaflets in systole, restore full leaflet motion, prevent progressive annular dilatation by inserting an annuloplasty ring and to ensure that on completion of the repair only a 'trace to mild' amount of mitral regurgitation remains.

Mitral valve repair is associated with an intra-operative mortality of 3% [10], although this figure may approach nearer 1% in experienced high volume centres [14].

Recurrence of mitral regurgitation may occur in upto 30% of patients [15]. The annual re-operation rate after initial repair to treat recurrent mitral regurgitation is 0.5-1.5% [16].

MVP may represent a large proportion of the caseload for percutaneous mitral valve leaflet technologies in the future.

Rheumatic Mitral Valve Disease

Mitral regurgitation may result from rheumatic heart disease although mitral stenosis or mixed mitral valve disease is more common. The incidence of rheumatic mitral valve disease has decreased in recent years in developed countries.

Examination of the mitral valve shows that the leaflets are thickened by fibrous tissue and a degree of calcification. Thickening and fusion of the chordae tendinae are also seen.

Ischaemic Mitral Regurgitation

Ischaemic mitral regurgitation results from sequlae of coronary artery disease. Acute myocardial ischaemia may result in transient dysfunction of the subvalvular apparatus or, more commonly, previous myocardial infarction may cause permanent dysfunction to the subvalvular apparatus. Mitral valve leaflets are structurally normal.

Generally the outcome for patients with ischaemic mitral regurgitation is worse than for those patients with similarly severe regurgitation from another cause. This is due to the superimposed ventricular dysfunction and volume overload.

Acute ischaemia may result in papillary muscle rupture or displacement, or annular dilatation due to left ventricular dilatation.

In the case of acute papillary muscle rupture urgent mitral valve surgery with revasularization is required. For those with papillary muscle dysfunction or annular dilatation, management may involve, haemodynamic support and observation with surgery being considered if there is no improvement.

In chronic ischaemic mitral regurgitation the case for surgery is less clear cut. Simultaneous Mitral Valve Replacement or mitral valve annuloplasty plus Coronary Artery Bypass Grafting may be considered.

Efficacy of percutaneous leaflet technologies in functional mitral regurgitation is less well established than in isolated prolpase.

Other Conditions

Miscellaneous conditions such as hypertrophic cardiomyopathy, dilated cardiomyopathy, ankylosing spondylitis and mucopolysaccharidoses can all be associated with mitral regurgitation.

MANAGEMENT OF MITRAL REGURGITATION

Regular electrocardiography, primarily to assess the cardiac rhythm, and echocardiography should be performed in all patients with mitral regurgitation. Transthoracic echocardiography allows assessment of the mechanism of mitral regurgitation, enables grading of it's severity and can assess the left ventricular size and function.

A semiquanitive scale is used to grade mitral regurgitation: grade I (mild), grade II (moderate), grade III (moderately severe) and grade IV (severe). Doppler assessments are recommended to define severe mitral reurgitation more precisely. In severe mitral regurgitation there is a regurgitant volume of 60ml or more, a regurgitant fraction of at least 50% and an effective regurgitant orifice of at least 40mm [2,17].

Asymptomatic patients with mitral regurgitation of grades I and II with no evidence of left ventricular dilatation or dysfunction should be observed.

Patients with severe mitral regurgitation with symptoms (breathlessness[New York Heart Association Class III], chest pain, syncope) or with evidence of left ventricular dysfunction (ejection fraction of less than 50%) or dilatation (Left Ventricular End Systolic Dimension >45mm) should be considered for surgery [9]. Asymptomatic patients with atrial fibrillation or pulmonary hypertension should be referred for consideration of intervention.

Mitral valve surgery may not be advisable in patients with significant respiratory, hepatic or renal dysfunction. Patients with marked peripheral vascular or cerebral arterial disease may also not be suitable. Although depressed myocardial function is associated with poor outcomes it is not a contra-indication to mitral valve surgery. The EUROSORE [18] or Society of Thoracic Surgeons risk calculator may be used to determine the best course of action.

The Percutaneous Approach

Percutaneous therapy to the mitral valve has been in development for over a quarter of a century. The first procedure ever attempted being balloon valvuloplasty for mitral stenosis in 1984 [19].

Therapies for mitral regurgitation have been more evasive. Several options are available which follow similar approaches to their well established surgical counterparts. These include leaflet repair, coronary sinus annuloplasty, direct annuloplasty, ventricular and atrial remodeling, valve replacement and chordal repair and implanation. The majority of these remain investigational.

Leaflet Technology

Surgical mitral valve replacement/repair has been the definitive treatment for severe mitral regurgitation for several decades. In certain patient groups, such as those with severe left ventricular dysfunction or co-morbidities which are associated with a high surgical risk, surgery may not be an option. The percutaneous technologies negate the use of cardiopulmonary bypass and sternotomy and offer an alternative approach to this high risk group.

It is possible, to engineer a double orifice, within the mitral valve, by suturing the free edges of the anterior and posterior leaflets, at mid point, percutaneously. A technique first described by Alfieri in 1990. This procedure may be suitable for patients with mitral regurgitation resulting from central malcoaptation of the valve. Currently more complicated leaflet repair is beyond the scope of interventional cardiologists.

When this technique is used during open heart surgery it is common practice to deploy an annuloplasty ring simultaneously. This is not currently the case in percutaneous procedures and the benefit, if any, to the addition of an annuloplasty ring is debated.

There are two devices with different modus operandi available.

The first is the Mobius device made by Edwards Lifesciences. This device uses a transeptal suction catheter to secure the mitral valve leaflets and deploy percutaneous sutures. Feasibility trials in animals and humans proved unsatisfactory and currently this technique is not being further developed.

The second is the Mitraclip made by Evalve. A multiaxel transeptal catheter facilitates the use of a metallic clip to grasp the two free edges of the anterior and posterior leaflets and join them. Transoesophageal Echocardiography guides the deployment and is used to assess the valve throughout the procedure. Clips can be removed if not satisfactory without injury to the leaflets or subvalvular structure. This means the physician can optomise the reduction in mitral regurgitation by trialing several points along the line of coaptation. Transoesophageal echocardiography enables functional assessment of the valve and the degree of regurgitation.

Alternatively if the physician is unable to deploy the Mitraclip with satisfactory results the device can be removed entirely and the patient considered for conventional surgical options. The design of the Mitraclip does not preclude surgical therapies even if left in place.

It is also possible to deploy an additional clip if required.

The EValve Mitraclip was granted a CE mark for the treatment of mitral regurgitation in Europe in September 2008.

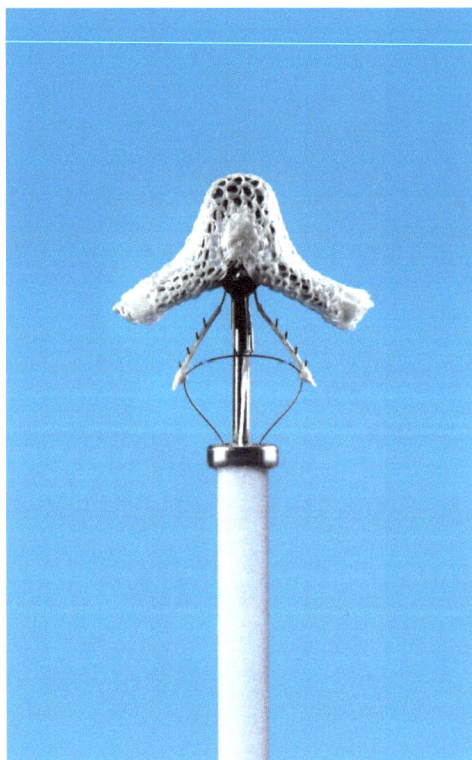

Figure 2: The EValve Mitraclip.

From the trial data available the Mitraclip is found to be effective and safe. It is the only leaflet device being used in clinical practice at present.

The phase I feasibility trial (Endovascular Valve Edge-to-Edge REpair Study [EVERSET] I) of Mitraclip included patients with functional or degenerative mitral regurgitation of grade 3 or above. Patients with rheumatic mitral regurgitation and severe left ventricular dysfunction (Ejection Fraction <25% or Left Ventricular End Systolic Diameter >55mm) were excluded. The Mitraclip was implanted in 42 of these patients. In 74% of patients the mitral regurgitation grade was reduced to grade 2 or below at time of discharge. Echocardiographic follow up of 22 of the patients who were discharged with a clip showed that this reduction was maintained at 6 month follow up [20].

The first large randomised trial comparing the Mitraclip to conventional surgery, EVEREST II, has finished recruiting and is expected to report on 2010. Approximately 300 patients with MR of grade 3 or above were randomized in a 2:1 ratio to percutaneous Mitraclip implantation or surgical mitral valve repair/replacement. Patients with severe left ventricular dysfunction and/or annular dilatation were excluded meaning the trial will assess structural valve disease.

Of 107 patients, who were in EVEREST I and the roll-in group of EVEREST II, acute procedural success was achieved in 74%(79/107). Mitral regurgitation was reduced at discharge to ≤grade 1 in 64% (51/79). This related to real clinical improvement of New York Heart Association class. Kaplan-Meier freedom from death and freedom from surgery at 3 years was 90.1% and 76.3% respectively [21].

Moreover the procedural success rates increased with the operators experience and adverse outcomes were minimal. There was one non-procedural in-hospital death. Partial clip detachment occurred in 9% of cases (ie detachment from one of the two valve leaflets). No cases of clip embolisation were reported. Other theoraectical complications include; complications from vascular access, cardiac tamponade from attempted transseptal puncure, atrial septal defect and iatrogenic mitral valve stenosis.

One limitation is that the majority of the patients in the EVEREST registry had mitral valve prolapse. It remains to be seen whether this technique will have the same success in patients with functional mitral regurgitation (defined as mitral regurgitation in the presence of echocardiographically 'normal' leaflets) although the available limited subcohort analysis of 23 patients is promising. Acute procedural success with residual mitral regurgitation of ≤grade 2 was achieved in 83%. Kaplan-Meirer freedom from death, mitral valve surgery and mitral regurgitation of >grade 2, at 3 years, is predicted as 64%.

The EVEREST II High Risk Registry recruited 78 patients symptomatic patients with mitral regurgitation of ≥grade 3 considered to be at high risk from conventional surgery [22]. The risk of surgical mortality was considered to be higher than 12% based on the patients Society of Transthoracic Surgeons risk model or a cardiac surgeons determination that the patient had at least one of the specified risk factors that resulted in at least 12% risk of surgical mortality. The average age or patients was 77 and most had several co-morbidites. 46 had functional mitral regurgitation and 32 had degenerative mitral regurgitation.

The acute procedural success rate was 96%. The mean predicted 30 day mortality (based on the sts score) of the group was 17.8%, however the actual figure was 7.7%. At 12 months, 74% of patients with matched data were in NYHA functional class I or II, compared to only 9% at baseline. This improvement in functional class was accompanied by improved left ventricular volumes and function.

The rate of hospitalization for heart failure in the year after treatment with the MitraClip system was significantly lower than the rate in the year prior to treatment.

Procedure

The National Institute of Clinical Excellence published guidance on the use of percutaneous valve technologies in August 2009 (IPG309). They have recommended that the procedure should only be used with special arrangements for clinical governance, consent and research for patients who are well enough for surgical mitral valve leaflet repair to treat their mitral regurgitation, or in the context of research patients who are not well enough for surgical mitral valve leaflet repair to treat their mitral regurgitation.

A team of interventional cardiologists, echocardiologists, anaesthetists, catheter laboratory technicians and nurses and echo technicians are needed.

A 24 French gauge guide catheter is inserted into the left atrium *via* a standard transseptal approach from the right femoral vein. The clip delivery system with the Mitraclip attached is then passed through the guide catheter. The clip is a polyester-covered device that can be opened and closed to grasp the leaflets on their atrial surface. Once the leaflets are captured and a double orifice has been created the device can be closed and then locked if the mitral regurgitation reduction is adequate.

The procedure is performed under general anaesthetic with transoesphageal echocardiography guidance.

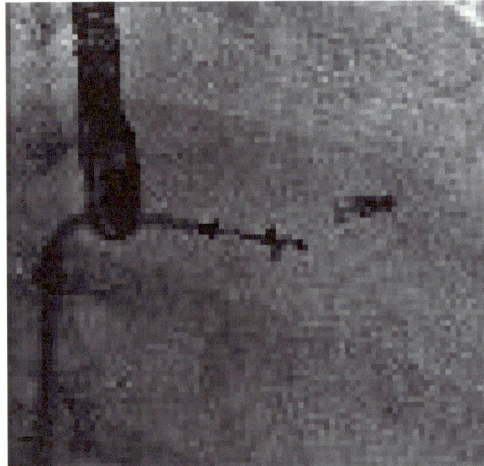

Figure 3: The Mitraclip has been deployed and is seen towards the right hand side of the image. The TOE probe and the delivery device are also evident.

The average length of hospital stay is 2 days. There is usually no requirement for a stay on the Intensive Care Unit. The proposed cost per patient is approximately £23,000. The average cost per patient with Mitral Regurgitation per annum to NHS is currently between £6,000 and £11,000.

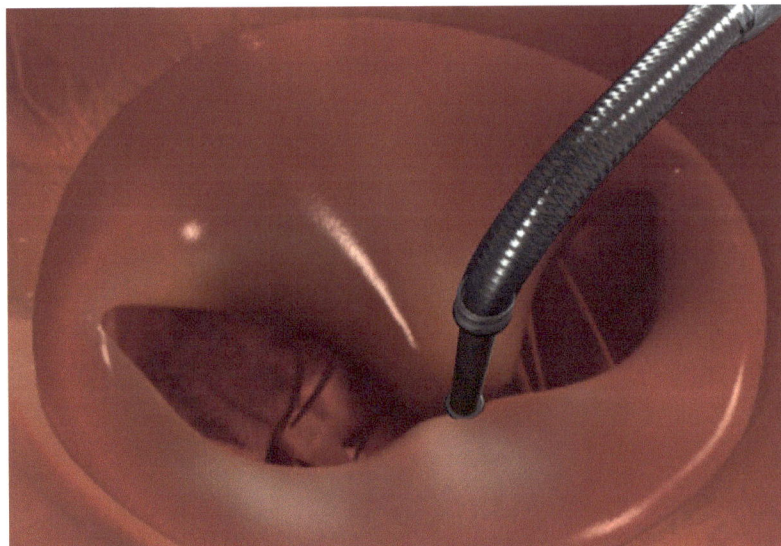

Figure 4: Double-orifice technique.

Efficacy and Safety of this Procedure

Very little is known at present about the long term success of percutaneous mitral valve repair and the implications of repair on later mitral valve surgery.

The risks that have been identified to date are those of Transoesophageal echocardiography, general anaesthetic, failure to implant the device (approximately 10%), complications from venous access, risk of trans-septal puncture, device embolisation, risk of thrombosis and stroke, recurrent mitral regurgitation and risk of infection. With the experience to date and the evidence currently available, the risks of these various potential complications has been small.

It seems inevitable that in the ensuing years we will see an expansion of the use of 'leaflet' technologies to treat mitral regurgitation in patients using a percutaneous approach.

REFERENCES

[1]   Avierinos JF, Inamo J, Grigioni F, *et al.* Sex differences in morphology and outcomes of mitral valve prolapse. Ann Intern Med 2008; 149: 787-95.

[2]   Hayek E, Gring CN, Griffin BP. Mitral valve prolapse. Lancet 2005; 365(9458): 507–18.

[3]   Barlow JB, Bosman CK. Aneurysmal protrusion of the posterior leaflet of the mitral valve. An auscultatory-electrocardiographic syndrome. Am Heart J 1966; 71(2): 166–78.

[4]   Barlow JB, Pocock WA. Mitral valve prolapse, the specific billowing mitral leaflet syndrome, or an insignificant non-ejection systolic click. Am Heart J 1979; 97: 277-85.

[5]   Ling LH, Enriquez-Sarano M, Seward JB, *et al.* Clinical outcome of mitral regurgitation due to flail leaflet. N Eng J Med 1996; 335: 1417-23.

[6]   Emond M, Mock MB, Davis KB, *et al.* Long-term survival of medically treated patients in the Coronary Artery Surgery Study (CASS) Registry. Circulation 1994; 90: 2645-2657.

[7]   Shuhaiber J, Anderson RJ. Meta-analysis of clinical outcomes following surgical mitral valve repair or replacement. Eur J Cardiothorac Surg 2007; 31: 267-275.

[8]   Grigioni F, Tribouilloy C, Avierinos JF, *et al.* Outcomes in mitral regurgitation due to flail leaflets: a multicenter European study. JACC Cardiovasc Imaging 2008; 1: 133-41.

[9]   American College of Cardiology, American Heart Association Task Force on Practice Guidelines. ACC/AHA 2006 guidelines for the management of patients with valvular heart disease: a report of the American College of Cardiology/American Heart Association Task Force on Practice Guidelines (Writing Committee to revise the 1998 guidelines for the management of patients with valvular heart disease) developed in collaboration with the Society of Cardiovascular Anesthesiologists endorsed by the Society for Cardiovascular Angiography and Interventions and the Society of Thoracic Surgeons. J Am Coll Cardiol 2006; 48: e1-e148.

[10]   Gillinov AM, Cosgrove DM III, Blackstone EH, *et al.* Durability of mitral valve repair for degenerative disease. J Thorac Cardiovasc Surg 1998; 116: 734-743.

[11]   Duran CG, Pomar JL, Revuelta JM, *et al.* Conservative operation for mitral insufficiency: critical analysis supported by postoperative hemodynamic studies of 72 patients. J Thorac Cardiovasc Surg 1980; 79: 326-337.

[12]   Mesana TG, Ibrahim M, Kulik A, *et al.* The "hybrid flip-over" technique for anterior leaflet prolapse repair. Ann Thorac Surg 2007; 83: 322-323.

[13]   Mesana T, Ibrahim M, Hynes M. A technique for annular placation to facilitate sliding plasty after extensive mitral valve posterior leaflet resection. Ann Thorac Surg 2005; 79: 720-722.

[14]   Gammie JS, O'Brien SM, Griffith BP, Ferguson TB, Peterson ED. Influence of hospital procedural volume on care process and mortality for patients undergoing elective surgery for mitral regurgitation. Circulation 2007; 115: 881-887.

[15]   Filsoufi F, Carpentier A. Principles of reconstructive surgery in degenerative mitral valve disease. Semin Thorac Cardiovasc Surg 2007; 19: 103-110.

[16]   Lee EM, Shapiro LM, Wells FC. Superiority of mitral valve repair in surgery for degenerative mitral regurgitation. Eur Heart J 1997; 18: 655-663.

[17]   Zoghbi WA, Enriquez-Sarano M, Foster E, *et al.* Recommendations for evaluation of the severity of native valvular regurgitation with two-dimensional and Doppler echocardiography. J Am Soc Echocardiogr 2003; 16: 777-802.

[18]   Nashef SA, Roques F, Michael P, *et al.* European system for cardiac operative risk evaluation (EuroSCORE). Eur J Cardiothorac Surg. 1999 Jul; 16(1): 9-13.

[19]   Inoue K, Owaki T, Nakamura T, *et al.* Clinical application of transvenous mitral commissurotomy by a new balloon catheter. J Thorac Cardiovasc Surg. 1984; 87: 394-402.

[20]   Herrmann HC, Feldman T. Percutaneous mitral valve edge-to-edge repair with the Evalve Mitraclip System: rationale and phase 1 results. Euro Intervention Supplements 2006; 1(suppl A): A36-9.

[21]   Feldman T, Kar S, Rinaldi M, *et al.* Percutaneous mitral valve repair with the Mitraclip system: safety and midterm durability in the initial EVEREST (Endovascular Valve Edge-to-Edge REpair Study) cohort. J Am Coll Cardiol, 2009; 54: 686-694.

[22]   Kar S. Experience with Mitraclip therapy in EVEREST II high-risk registry. EURO PCR 2009.

CHAPTER 6

Percutaneous Mitral Annuloplasty

Liam M McCormick[1],* and Michael O'Sullivan[2]

[1]Papworth Hospital, Cambridge, UK and [2]Papworth Hospital, Cambridge, UK

Abstract: Functional Mitral Regurgitation (MR), due to incomplete mitral leaflet closure rather than an inherent abnormality in the valve apparatus, is a highly prevalent condition that is associated with an adverse prognosis in patients with heart failure. To date, traditional medical therapies have largely been ineffective, and enthusiasm for various surgical strategies has been limited by their lack of prognostic benefit and perceived high risk. In order to overcome some of these issues, a number of percutaneous approaches have recently emerged, and while these techniques are still in the research arena, there is already encouraging early data. This chapter will address the pathophysiologal mechanisms involved in functional MR, and summarise the current data available on percutaneous mitral valve therapies, with a particular emphasis on devices involving 'indirect annuloplasty' via the coronary sinus.

Mitral Regurgitation

Valvular heart disease is an important public health problem, with moderate to severe lesions affecting 2.5% of the general population. Mitral regurgitation (MR) is the most common of these valvulopathies, with a prevalence of 15.7% in those older than 64 years of age [1]. Inmpetence of the mitral valve may be due to abnormalities in any of the structures that constitute the valve apparatus - namely the leaflets, chordae tendinae, papillary muscles, or mitral annulus. In broad terms, the aetiology of MR can be classified as either:

1. Organic - when it is secondary to structural alterations of the mitral or subvalvar apparatus, such as degenerative (including mitral valve prolapse) and rheumatic disease, infective endocarditis and annular calcification.

2. Functional – when it occurs in the setting of structurally normal valve leaflets and chordae, usually secondary to alterations in left ventricular (LV) geometry that occur with myocardial ischaemia or non-ischaemic cardiomyopathy.

This chapter will focus on only functional mitral regurgitation.

Functional Mitral Regurgitation

Functional MR is due to incomplete mitral leaflet closure that occurs as a secondary process, rather than due to an inherent abnormality in the valve apparatus [2]. Proposed pathophysiological mechanisms for this process include global LV dysfunction decreasing the ventricular force acting to close the leaflets, dilatation of the mitral annulus, and alterations in LV geometry at the site from which the papillary muscles arise [3]. Whilst it is likely that all 3 factors play a role, experimental studies have demonstrated that the predominant mechanism is probably apical displacement of the papillary muscles with tenting of the leaflets away from the annulus and subsequent incomplete leaflet coaptation [4].

Functional MR is an important entity because it is frequently found in patients with impaired LV systolic function and in this group, has been shown to be associated with an adverse prognosis. Robbins *et al.* retrospectively investigated a group of patients with a clinical diagnosis of heart failure, and demonstrated that in patients with an ejection fraction (EF) ≤ 40%, moderate to severe MR was present in 59% (74% of inpatients and 45% of outpatients). When these patients were compared with those without MR or with mild MR, there was a significantly higher mortality rate in the moderate to severe group (39% vs 19%) at mean follow-up of 47 ± 19 months [5].

Koelling *et al.* reviewed the clinical and echocardiographic characteristics of 1421 consecutive patients who were found to have LV dysfunction (EF ≤ 35%). Moderate MR was found in 18.9% of patients, and severe MR in 29.7%. Over the average 1 year follow-up period, severe MR was an independent predictor of mortality and conveyed an 84% additional risk of death. Furthermore, there was an incremental risk of death with increasing grades of MR.

*Address correspondence to Liam M McCormick:** Papworth Hospital, Cambridge, UK; E-mail: Liam.McCormick@papworth.nhs.uk

Peter M. Schofield (Ed)

This study demonstrated therefore that MR is common in patients with LV systolic dysfunction, and its severity is highly predictive of an adverse prognosis [6].

Several studies have reported on the association between ischaemic heart disease and MR. In a 10-year cohort study, Bursi *et al.* investigated the prevalence and prognostic impact of MR in 773 patients who underwent an echocardiogram within 30 days of an incident myocardial infarction. MR was found in 50% of patients (mild in 38% and moderate or severe in 12%) but interestingly, a murmur was only detected clinically in approximately half of these. After a mean of 4.7 ± 3.3 years of follow-up, MR was associated with a > 3-fold excess risk of heart failure and similarly, the presence of moderate to severe MR was independently associated with a 55% increased risk of death. The risk of heart failure and death exhibited a graded "dose-response" relationship with the severity of MR, which may suggest a causal relationship [7].

Grigioni *et al.* investigated 173 asymptomatic or minimally symptomatic (New York Heart Association functional (NYHA) class I or II) patients who underwent echocardiography > 16 days after myocardial infarction. When compared with those without MR, patients with MR were found to have significantly higher rates of the combined end-point of congestive heart failure or death (69% vs 30%) at 5 years of follow-up. They also found that more severe degrees of MR, as assessed by effective regurgitant orifices were independently associated with higher event rates, in support of a degree-effect relationship [8].

Medical Management

Currently, there are limited effective therapeutic options available for patients with functional MR. Medical therapy is established as first-line treatment for patients with LV systolic dysfunction, and should be optimised before consideration of more invasive options [9, 10]. There is some data to suggest that medical therapy may reduce regurgitant volumes in patients with functional MR, but it is likely that its primary effect is on treatment of the antecedent heart failure. Beta-blockers and ACE inhibitors effect inverse geometric ventricular remodelling and should help to restore the normal orientation of the papillary muscles to the annulus. Whilst Carvedilol has been shown to reduce the severity of functional MR [11], the evidence for ACE inhibition is not as strong. Vasodilators (e.g. nitroprusside, long acting nitrates, hydralazine) in association with loop diuretics, may also reduce the severity of MR in selected patients but it is unlikely that they confer any significant long-term prognostic benefit [12]. Since functional MR is strongly associated with LV dilatation and dyssynchrony, a subset of patients with an increased QRS duration will be candidates for cardiac resynchronisation therapy (CRT). CRT has been shown to improve LV function and in doing so, can reduce the severity of functional MR both acutely and chronically [13]. This occurs as a result of partially reversed LV remodelling, decreased effective regurgitant orifice area and realignment of contractile timing of the papillary muscles.

Surgery for Functional Mitral Regurgitation

Standard surgical therapy for functional MR involves annuloplasty with a ring that is designed to correct annular dilatation, restore leaflet coaptation, and reduce effective regurgitant orifice area [3]. However, mitral valve surgery in this setting is a controversial issue. It is clear that chronic volume overload contributes to progressive ventricular remodelling, which in turn begets progressive MR. As such, surgical correction may in theory break the cycle, but may not confer any significant benefit if the adverse ventricular remodelling is irreversible. Furthermore, the perceived operative risk is not insignificant in these patients, and there have been realistic concerns regarding the deleterious effects of increased afterload on an already failing ventricle [14]. Data on the results of surgery are limited and it is difficult to draw conclusions from series involving small numbers of patients with varying degrees of revascularisation. Furthermore, there has never been a prospective randomised trial comparing medical therapy with mitral valve surgery in this population, and no trials have compared different techniques of mitral valve repair, or mitral valve repair with mitral valve replacement.

Despite the inherent difficulties in drawing strong conclusions from a group of small retrospective, observational studies that are mostly single centre, several themes appear to be consistent:

- In experienced centres, surgery is feasible with acceptable perioperative mortality rates that vary from 3 to 6% [15,16,17,18,19] 5-year survival appears to range from 60 to 78% [15, 16, 18, 19] but patient populations within the series have varied significantly with respect to aetiology (ischaemic vs. idiopathic), ejection fraction, proportion undergoing concomitant revascularisation and surgical techniques used.

- Most patients who undergo surgery have statistically significant improvements in NYHA functional class [15, 16, 17, 19, 20, 21, 22], exercise capacity and quality of life.

- Some, but not all series have reported on positive functional outcomes such as reverse remodelling (e.g. improvement in LVEF [20, 21, 22], reductions in end-diastolic and end-systolic volumes [17, 20, 22].

Despite these seemingly encouraging results, no study has demonstrated any mortality benefit of mitral valve repair or replacement over conventional medical or device therapies. There are a number of potential reasons for this:

1. By definition, patients with functional MR have significantly impaired LV function which translates to a high surgical risk. It may be that any potential benefit conferred from surgical correction of MR is counterbalanced by peri-operative mortality rates.

2. Severe MR in the setting of advanced LV dysfunction represents a "ventricular problem", and this may dictate overall prognosis [23]. If the valvular incompetence is only a marker of a poor ventricle, correction of this secondary pathology alone may not be sufficient to confer prognostic benefit.

3. There is a high rate of recurrence after surgery. Significant (moderate to severe) MR recurs in as many as 30% of patients within 12 months [24] and is thought to be due to progressive LV remodelling particularly involving the posterior wall [25].

4. A blunderbuss approach of operating on all patients with functional MR may not be effective. As with any assessment of candidacy for cardiac surgery, patient selection is vital and there may be specific cohorts of patients who would benefit over and above the general population. It would seem sensible that this selection process involves careful consideration of peri-operative risk and evidence of LV reverse remodeling viability [26].

5. Surgical trials are poor. There are no randomized controlled trials comparing surgery with medical or device therapy, and as yet, there is no evidence that surgery for patients with functional MR and advanced LV dysfunction prolongs life.

So how does one make strong recommendations based on the limited and somewhat confusing information that is currently available? The European Society of Cardiology suggests that "isolated mitral valve surgery in combination with LV reconstruction techniques may be considered in selected patients with severe functional MR and severely depressed LV function, including those with coronary disease, where bypass surgery is not indicated, who remain symptomatic despite optimal medical therapy, and if co-morbidity is low, the aim being to avoid or postpone transplantation. In the other patients, medical therapy followed by transplantation when this fails is probably the best option. However, surgery on the regurgitant mitral valve should not be considered in 'in extremis patients' with low output, severe right ventricular failure, and high co-morbidity." [9]

The lack of a clear surgical strategy for the mechanical treatment of functional MR, and the perceived high surgical risk, has fuelled interest in minimally invasive / percutaneous approaches.

PERCUTANEOUS APPROACHES TO MITRAL REGURGITATION

Over recent years, a number of percutaneous therapies for MR have emerged as clinicians look to bypass the risks and controversial issues associated with surgery. Technological advances have facilitated the development of numerous devices which typically mirror established surgical techniques. These devices aim to address the various pathophysiological mechanisms involved in the regurgitant mitral valve - annular dilatation, impaired leaflet mobility and coaptation, and LV remodelling with apical displacement of papillary muscles and subsequent tethering and tenting of leaflets. The currently available technologies can be classified as follows:

1. Annuloplasty Devices

    - Indirect *via* the coronary sinus (e.g. MONARC, CARILLON, PTMA)

    - Direct annuloplasty (e.g. Mitralign, Guided Delivery System, QuantumCor)

2.   Leaflet Repair Devices (e.g. Mitraclip)

3.   Chamber Remodelling Devices (e.g. Coapsys, PS3)

This chapter will focus on the percutaneous approach to mitral valve annuloplasty. For further information on leaflet repair devices, see Chapter 5.

Indirect Annuloplasty *via* the Coronary Sinus

The mitral annulus is an elliptical "D-shaped" structure composed of a fibrous connective tissue ring called the annulus fibrosa. The anterior component is straight and forms part of the aortic-mitral junction. The posterior portion is C-shaped and in direct continuity with the muscular fibres of the atrial and ventricular walls [27]. Whilst the anterior portion is virtually impossible to deform *via* a percutaneous approach, there are a number of structural characteristics of the posterior component which make it an attractive target for indirect annuloplasty. Firstly, the posterior mitral valve leaflet has hinge lines on both its atrial and ventricular surfaces. This is in contrast to the anterior mitral valve leaflet, in which the ventricular surface is in direct fibrous continuity with the left and non-coronary cusps of the aortic valve. Secondly, the posterior mitral annulus is composed of considerably less fibrous tissue, rendering it weaker than its anterior counterpart. Thirdly, the posterior annulus is in close proximity to the atrioventricular groove and coronary sinus, which make it anatomically accessible *via* a transvenous approach.

The cardiac venous system demonstrates considerable anatomical variability [28]. In most people, the anterior interventricular vein runs parallel to the left anterior descending artery in the anterior interventricular groove, and joins the great cardiac vein which runs laterally along the left atrioventricular groove. At the point where it merges with the oblique left atrial vein, the great cardiac vein becomes the coronary sinus, which empties into the inferoposteromedial aspect of the right atrium. The middle cardiac vein runs parallel to the posterior descending artery in the posterior interventricular groove, and drains into the coronary sinus [28]. The coronary sinus ostium is usually marked by the presence of the Thebesius valve which can obstruct cannulation. The most consistent features of the cardiac venous anatomy are the coronary sinus, great cardiac vein and middle cardiac vein, whereas the left marginal and posterior LV branches of the great cardiac vein are the most variable [28].

Surgical mitral annuloplasty with an undersized ring that encircles the entire mitral valve causes compression of the mitral annulus and leaflets along the septal to lateral axis. This results in improved leaflet coaptation and a reduced regurgitant orifice, with a subsequent reduction in miral regurgitation. As discussed earlier in this chapter, the surgical approach can lead to an improvement in symptoms and LV function, but there are still real doubts over its effect on overall prognosis, and the risks of morbidity and mortality are significant. Percutaneous mitral annuloplasty aims to mimic the traditional surgical technique through a less invasive approach, with the potential for reduced procedural risk. As such, it appears to be a particularly attractive option for patients with comorbidities or less severe MR.

However, despite its obvious appeal, there are a number of potential problems with the indirect coronary sinus approach to percutaneous mitral annulopasty:

•   The coronary sinus is only in contact with the posterior aspect of the mitral annulus, and therefore, annuloplasty *via* this system may not be as effective as the surgical alternative which involves placing an undersized ring that encircles the entire mitral valve.

•   There is considerable variability in the horizontal and vertical relation of the coronary sinus to the mitral valve annulus. Tops *et al.* reported that the coronary sinus is located superior to the mitral annulus in 90% and 54% of patients at its mid and proximal segments respectively [29]. As such, mitral annular deformation may occur suboptimally from secondary tension effects from the left atrial wall [27].

•   The left circumflex coronary artery courses between the coronary sinus and mitral annulus in 64% to 81% of the population [30,31]. Therefore, coronary sinus annuoplasty devices in these patients are associated with a real risk of arterial compression and myocardial infarction [32].

•   By definition, patients with functional MR have impaired LV function, and so a significant proportion of these will be candidates for percutaneous mitral annuloplasty as well as CRT. As the coronary sinus is used for LV lead placement in CRT devices, patients who have undergone this therapy may not be suitable for indirect annuloplasty.

- There is a theoretical risk of coronary sinus thrombosis and erosion, although neither of these complications has been reported to date.

Edwards MONARC System

The Edwards MONARC device is a second-generation implant, the structure of which is based upon the Edwards Viking annuloplasty system [27]. The Viking device is made up of 2 self-expandable nitinol (nickel-titanium alloy) anchors connected by a spring-like bridge segment. The distal anchor is deployed in the great cardiac vein with the proximal anchor deployed in the proximal coronary sinus. The bridge has memory properties which results in shortening at body temperature. This has the effect of anterior displacement of the posterior mitral annulus, with reductions in mitral annulus diameter and septal-lateral distance. Webb *et al.* have reported their first-in-man experience with the Viking system [33]. Four patients with chronic ischaemic MR (grade 2 – 4) underwent successful implantation of the device. In one further patient, implantation was unsuccessful due to perforation of the anterior interventricular vein with subsequent pericardial effusion. In the 4 successfully implanted patients, average grade of MR was reduced from 3.0 to 1.6. However, this benefit was not sustained because of device failure in 3 patients caused by separation of the bridge from the anchor within 3 months of implant.

The second-generation MONARC device has overcome the structural short-comings associated with the Viking system, with no further reports of device separation. The bridge connecting the two anchors consists of biodegradable spacers which dissolve in the first few weeks after implant. This allows the bridge to shorten by as much as 30% of its original length, and results in cinching of the mitral annulus [34]. The EVOLUTION I trial evaluated the safety of the re-engineered MONARC device in 72 patients with dilated or ischaemic cardiomyopathy and functional MR [35]. Successful implantation occurred in 59 patients (82%) and at 2 years follow-up, 72% of patients were free of major adverse cardiac events. Only 6 of the 16 events were felt to be device or procedure-related with 2 cardiac tamponades (possibly secondary to use of a non-J-tipped guidewire), 3 myocardial infarctions (due to compression of a coronary artery) and 1 death (as a result of LV failure after one of the aforementioned myocardial infarctions).

Available efficacy analysis in 21 patients at 2 year follow up has demonstrated that 54.5% of patients have had at least one grade reduction in MR, although the proportion of responders is higher for those with more severe MR at baseline (*i.e.* response rate is 80% in patients with grade 3 or 4 MR). Furthermore, there has been a statistically significant improvement in NYHA functional class, and favourable changes in physiological parameters associated with LV remodelling (e.g. EF, end-diastolic and end-systolic volumes) [35]. Encouragingly, there appears to be little deterioration in quantitative assessments of MR from 1 to 2 years. These preliminary data therefore demonstrate early feasibility, safety and durability of the MONARC percutaneous annuloplasty device, and recruitment has already commenced for a larger EVOLUTION II trial to focus more attention on efficacy and clinical outcome measures.

Cardiac Dimensions CARILLON Mitral Contour System Device

The Carillon device consists of distal and proximal nitinol-based anchors that are separated by a metal bridge. The anchors are double helices with shape memory characteristics that are delivered into the coronary sinus *via* the internal jugular vein through a titanium crimping tube [27]. After the distal anchor is deployed in the great cardiac vein, manual tension is applied to the system which results in plication, or cinching, of the mitral annulus. As there is an immediate shortening of the coronary sinus, and subsequent cinching of the mitral annulus, deployment of the device can be guided by echocardiographic measures of MR reduction. Importantly, and unlike the MONARC system, the CARILLON device is fully retrievable upto final release. As such, the anchors can be recaptured by releasing traction if there is concern regarding coronary artery compression, haemodynamic compromise, displacement of the distal anchor, or insufficient reduction in MR [27].

The AMADEUS trial evaluated the feasibility and safety of the CARILLON device in 48 patients with dilated or ischaemic cardiomyopathy (EF < 40%), moderate to severe functional MR and NYHA class II – IV symptoms [36]. Eighteen patients did not have the device implanted due to access issues, coronary artery compromise or insufficient reduction in MR. After 30 days, six patients suffered a total of 7 major adverse events – 1 coronary sinus dissection, 2 coronary sinus perforations (1 of these necessitating pericardial drainage), 3 subclinical myocardial infarctions (*i.e.* 3-fold increase in CK-MB without chest pain or ECG changes) and 1 death (as a result of acute on chronic renal failure due to contrast nephropathy in a patient who underwent coronary angiography the day after the procedure to investigate a post-procedural rise in cardiac enzymes).

Available efficacy analysis at 6 month follow-up in 24 patients who received the CARILLON device demonstrated statistically significant 23% average reduction in MR across 5 different echocardiographic parameters. There was also a significant reduction in mitral annulus diameter and a trend towards reduced LV end-diastolic volume. There was also a significant improvement in symptoms with the average NYHA classification reducing from 2.9 to 1.8. At baseline, 80% of patients were in NYHA class III or IV, whereas at 6 month follow-up, 88% were in NYHA class I or II. Similarly, there was a significant improvement in 6-minute walk distance and 84% of patients reported some degree of improved quality of life [36].

A second pilot study, the TITAN trial, has been designed to evaluate longer-term safety and efficacy (*i.e.* up to 5 years) of the CARILLON system in 53 patients [37]. At 30-day follow up, the only major adverse event was 1 death, with no incidences of myocardial infarction or coronary sinus complications. This significantly lower rate compared with the AMADEUS trial indicates a learning curve effect. Encouragingly, TITAN has also revealed a significant reduction in echocardiographic (*i.e.* degree of MR) and functional parameters (*i.e.* NYHA class, 6 minute walk test and quality of life). These preliminary data therefore demonstrate feasibility, safety and efficacy of the CARILLON Mitral Contour System device, and pave the way for the development of a randomised trial in a larger cohort of patients.

Viacor PTMA (Percutaneous Transvenous Mitral Annuloplasty) Device

The Viacor PTMA device consists of a polytetrafluoroethylene (PTFE) catheter that is delivered into the coronary sinus *via* the subclavian vein, with the distal tip seated in the anterior interventricular vein and the proximal hub left in a subclavicular pocket to enable further access at a later date [38]. The catheter contains 3 parallel lumens through which nitinol rods of varying stiffness, length and taper can be inserted. Unlike the previously mentioned annuloplasty devices, the Viacor PTMA device produces an outward force at its proximal and distal segments such that the midportion of the posterior mitral annulus is displaced anteriorly with subsequent reduction of the septal-lateral dimension and mitral regurgitant orifice [27]. As the number, stiffness and length of the rods can be varied with time, incremental modifications of the degree of tension, and hence mitral annular geometry, can be achieved.

The PTOLEMY I trial evaluated the feasibility and safety of the PTMA device in 27 symptomatic patients (NYHA class II – III) with impaired LV function (EF 20 - 50%) and moderate to severe functional MR [39]. Eight patients had a failed diagnostic procedure – 6 due to unsuccessful venous access, 1 due to guidewire perforation and 1 due to anatomical exclusion. Of the 19 patients who successfully completed the diagnostic PTMA procedure, 6 did not have sufficient reductions in MR and did not receive the device. The remaining 13 patients underwent attempted implantation of the PTMA system, and of these, 4 were unsuccessful – 2 due to device instability and 2 due to difficulties in device delivery. Of the 9 patients who successfully received the device, 4 were removed – 1 due to device fracture, and 3 due to referral for surgical annuloplasty. After 30 days, four patients suffered a total of 5 major adverse events – 1 pericardial effusion necessitating pericardiocentesis, 1 circumflex stent implantation due to acute vessel occlusion likely due to compression from the device, 1 device fracture (diagnosed on chest radiography) resulting in loss of efficacy but no clinical sequelae, 1 episode of transient renal dysfunction and 1 episode of pneumonia.

Available efficacy analysis in the 19 patients who underwent a successful diagnostic PTMA procedure demonstrated an acute reduction in MR grade (from 3.2 to 2.0). In those patients who underwent successful implantation of the device, an average sustained reduction of mitral annulus septal-lateral dimension by 4mm was observed at 3 months. [39]. In some patients, this reduction has been maintained for more than 1 year [40]. These preliminary data therefore demonstrate early feasibility and safety of the Viacor PTMA device, and recruitment has already commenced for a larger PTOLEMY II trial to focus more attention on efficacy and clinical outcome measures.

Direct Annuloplasty

Some of the limitations of the indirect coronary sinus approach can be overcome through direct percutaneous annuloplasty. A number of devices have been designed and are in the very early stages of development.

Mitralign Percutaneous Annuloplasty System

The Mitralign system operates *via* a retrograde transaortic valve approach. The 12.5 F guide catheter is delivered into the LV and positioned beneath the posterior mitral leaflet. Radiofrequency is used to penetrate a number of wires through the posterior annulus which are then anchored. The anchors are connected by a drawstring suture which can reduce the annular dimensions when tethered [38]. At the time of writing, this procedure had been performed in 4 patients, and 12 month follow-up data has demonstrated reductions in MR, end-systolic and end-diastolic LV volumes, and mitral valve area [41]. Although the concept is attractive, the technique is challenging and a simpler design has been developed to enable further evaluation in clinical trials.

Guided Delivery System

Similar to the Mitralign technique, a catheter is used to place multiple anchors in the mitral annulus, which can be tethered. At the time of writing, no human data are available [38].

QuantumCor Device

A novel approach to direct annuloplasty, and thus far only tested in animals, the QuantumCor device applies radiofrequency energy directly to the mitral annulus to cause fibrosis of collagen and shrinkage of the annulus [38].

CONCLUSION

Functional MR is highly prevalent and is associated with poor prognosis in patients with heart failure. Nonetheless, there is no widely accepted mechanical approach to the treatment of this problem, largely because of the risks and lack of prognostic benefit of surgery in this population. There is increasing interest in percutaneous approaches to the treatment of functional MR, with most techniques involving 'indirect annuloplasty' *via* the coronary sinus. Such techniques remain in the research arena, although there are encouraging early data. We are optimistic that percutaneous mitral annuloplasty will become part of standard clinical practice for highly selected patients within the next 3 years.

REFERENCES

[1]   Nkomo VT, Gardin JM, Skelton TN, Gottdiener JS, Scott CG, Enriquez-Sarano M. Burden of valvular heart diseases: a population-based study. Lancet 2006; 368: 1005-11.
[2]   Goldberg SL. Coronary sinus annuloplasty for mitral regurgitation. Cardiac Interventions Today. August/September 2009, 74 - 78.
[3]   Levine RA, Hung J, Otsuji Y, Messas E, Liel-Cohen N, Nathan N, Handschumacher MD, Guerrero JL, He S, Yoganathan AP, Vlahakes GJ. Mechanistic insights into functional mitral regurgitation. Curr Cardiol Rep 2002 Mar; 4(2): 125-9.
[4]   Levine RA, Schwammenthal E. Ischemic mitral regurgitation on the threshold of a solution: from paradoxes to unifying concepts. Circulation 2005; 112: 745–58.
[5]   Robbins JD, Maniar PB, Cotts W, Parker MA, Bonow RO, Gheorghiade M. Prevalence and Severity of Mitral Regurgitation in Chronic Systolic Heart Failure. Am J Cardiol 2003; 91: 360-2.
[6]   Koelling TM, Aaronson KD, Cody RJ, Bach DS, Armstrong WF. Prognostic significance of mitral regurgitation and tricuspid regurgitation in patients with left ventricular systolic dysfunction. Am Heart J. 2002; 144: 524–529.
[7]   Bursi F, Enriquez-Sarano M, Nkomo VT, Jacobsen SJ, Weston SA, Meverden RA, Roger VL. Heart Failure and Death after Myocardial Infarction in the Community. The Emerging Role of Mitral Regurgitation. Circulation 2005; 111: 295-301.
[8]   Grigioni F, Detaint D, Avierino JF, Scott C, Tajik J, Enriquez-Sarano M. Contribution of Ischaemic Mitral Regurgitation to Congestive Heart Failure after Myocardial Infarction. J Am Coll Cardiol 2005; 45: 260-7.
[9]   Vahanian A, Baumgartner H, Bax J, *et al.* Guidelines on the management of valvular heart disease. The Task Force on the Management of Valvular Heart Disease of the European Society of Cardiology. Eur Heart J 2007; 28: 230-68.
[10]   Bonow RO, Carabello BA, Chatterjee K, *et al.* ACC/AHA 2006 Guidelines for the Management of Patients with Valvular Heart Disease: A Report of the American College of Cardiology/American Heart Association Task Force on Practice Guidelines (Writing Committee to Revise the 1998 Guidelines for the Management of Patients With Valvular Heart Disease): Developed in Collaboration With the Society of Cardiovascular Anesthesiologists and the Society of Thoracic Surgeons: Endorsed by the Society for Cardiovascular Angiography and Interventions and the Society of Thoracic Surgeons. Circulation 2006; 114: e84-e231.
[11]   Lowes BD, Gill EA, Abraham WT, *et al.* Effects of carvedilol on left ventricular mass, chamber geometry, and mitral regurgitation in chronic heart failure. Am J Cardiol 1999; 83: 1201–5.

[12]   Kizilbash AM, Willett DL, Brickner ME, *et al.* Effects of afterload reduction on vena contracta width in mitral regurgitation. J Am Coll Cardiol 1998; 32: 427–31.

[13]   Auricchio A, Abraham WT. Cardiac resynchronization therapy: current state of the art. Circulation 2004; 109: 300 –7.

[14]   Phillips HR, Levine FH, Carter JE, Boucher CA, Osbakken MD, Okada RD, Akins CW, Daggett WM, Buckley MJ, Pohost GM. Mitral valve replacement for isolated mitral regurgitation: analysis of clinical course and late postoperative left ventricular ejection fraction. Am J Cardiol. 1981 Oct; 48(4): 647-54.

[15]   Calafiore AM, Di Mauro M, Gallina S, *et al.* Mitral valve surgery for chronic ischemic mitral regurgitation. Ann Thorac Surg 2004; 77: 1989–97.

[16]   Calafiore AM, Gallina S, Di Mauro M, *et al.* Mitral valve procedure in dilated cardiomyopathy: repair or replacement? Ann Thorac Surg 2001; 71: 1146 –53.

[17]   De Bonis M, Lapenna E, La Canna G, *et al.* Mitral valve repair for functional mitral regurgitation in end-stage dilated cardiomyopathy: role of the "edge-to-edge" technique. Circulation 2005; 112 Suppl 1: I402– 8

[18]   Wu AH, Aaronson KD, Bolling SF, Pagani FD, Welch K, Koelling TM. Impact of mitral valve annuloplasty on mortality risk in patients with mitral regurgitation and left ventricular systolic dysfunction. J Am Coll Cardiol 2005; 45: 381–7.

[19]   Mihaljevic T, Lam BK, Rajeswaran J, *et al.* Impact of mitral valve annuloplasty combined with revascularization in patients with functional ischemic mitral regurgitation. J Am Coll Cardiol 2007; 49: 2191–201.

[20]   Acker MA, Bolling S, Shemin R, *et al.* Mitral valve surgery in heart failure: insights from the Acorn clinical trial. J Thorac Cardiovasc Surgery 2006; 132: 568-77.

[21]   Chen FY, Adams DH, Aranki SF, Collins JJ Jr, Couper GS, Rizzo RJ, Cohn LH. Mitral valve repair in cardiomyopathy. Circulation. 1998 Nov 10; 98(19 Suppl): II124-7.

[22]   Bolling SF, Francis D. Pagani FD, Michael Deeb G, Bach DS. Intermediate-Term Outcome Of Mitral Reconstruction In Cardiomyopathy. J Thorac Cardiovasc Surg 1998; 115: 381-388.

[23]   Carabello B. The current therapy for mitral regurgitation. J Am Coll Cardiol 2008; 52: 319 –26.

[24]   McGee ED, Gillinov AM, Blackstone EH, *et al.* Recurrent mitral regurgitation after annuloplasty for functional ischemic mitral regurgitation. J Thorac Cardiovasc Surg 2004; 128: 916 –24.

[25]   Hung J, Papakostas L, Tahta SA, Hardy BG, Bollen BA, Duran CM, Levine RA. Mechanism of recurrent ischemic mitral regurgitation after annuloplasty. Continued LV remodeling as a moving target. Circulation. 2004; 110 [suppl II] : II-85–II-90.

[26]   Di Salvo TG, Acker MA, Dec GW, Byrne JG. Mitral valve surgery in advanced heart failure. J Am Coll Cardiol 2010; 55: 271–82.

[27]   Piazza N, Bonan R. Transcatheter mitral valve repair for functional mitral regurgitation: coronary sinus approach. J Interven Cardiol 2007; 20: 495–508.

[28]   Singh JP, Houser S, Heist EK, Ruskin JN. The coronary venous anatomy: a segmental approach to aid cardiac resynchronisation therapy. J. Am. Coll. Cardiol. 2005; 46; 68-74.

[29]   Tops LF, Van de Veire NR, Schuijf JD, *et al.* Noninvasive evaluation of coronary sinus anatomy and its relation to the mitral valve annulus: Implications for percutaneous mitral annuloplasty. Circulation 2007; 115: 1426–1432.

[30]   Maselli D, Guarracino F, Chiaramonti F, *et al.* Percutaneous mitral annuloplasty: An anatomic study of human coronary sinus and its relation with mitral valve annulus and coronary arteries. Circulation 2006; 114: 377–380.

[31]   Mao S, Shinbane JS, Girsky MJ, Child J, Carson S, Oudiz RJ, Budoff MJ. Coronary venous imaging whit electron beam computed tomographic angiography: three-dimensional mapping and relationship with coronary arteries. Am Heart J. 2005; 150: 315–322.

[32]   Maniu CV, Patel JB, Reuter DG, *et al.* Acute and chronic reduction of functional mitral regurgitation in experimental heart failure by percutaneous mitral annuloplasty. J Am Coll Cardiol 2004; 44: 1652–1661.

[33]   Webb JG, Harnek J, Munt BI, *et al.* Percutaneous transvenous mitral annuloplasty initial human experience with device implantation in the coronary sinus. Circulation 2006; 113: 851–855.

[34]   Masson JB, Webb JG. Percutaneous mitral annuloplasty. Coronary Artery Disease 2009; 20: 183-188.

[35]   Harnek J. September 22, 2009, 2-year Interim Results of the Percutaneous MONARC System for the Treatment of Functional Mitral Regurgitation (presented at TCT 2009).

[36]   Schofer J, Siminiak T, Haude M, Herrman JP, Vainer J, Wu JC, Levy WC, Mauri L, Feldman T, Kwong RY, Kaye DM, Duffy SJ, Tübler T, Degen H, Brandt MC, Van Bibber R, Goldberg S, Reuter DG, Hoppe UC. Percutaneous Mitral Annuloplasty for Functional Mitral Regurgitation. Results of the CARILLON Mitral Annuloplasty Device European Union Study. Circulation 2009; 120: 326-333.

[37]   Schofer J. September 25, 2009, Results with Acute Tensioning. From AMADEUS and TITAN to a US pivotal Randomised Trial (Cardiac Dimensions CARILLON) (presented at TCTMD).

[38]   Alqoofi F, Feldman T. Percutaneous Approaches to Mitral Regurgitation. Curr Treat Options Cardiovasc Med 2009; 11: 476-482.

[39] Sack S, Kahlert P, Bilodeau L, *et al.* Percutaneous Transvenous Mitral Annuloplasty. Initial Human Experience with a Novel Coronary Sinus Implant Device. Circ Cardiovasc Intervent 2009; 2: 277-284).

[40] Bilodeau L. September 25, 2009, Results with Adjustable Nitinol Rods. From PTOLEMY I to PTOLEMY II (presented at TCT 2009).

[41] Buellesfeld L. September, 2009, Mitralign: From Trident to Bident. Clinical Trial Update (presented at TCT 2009).

CHAPTER 7

The Use of Left Atrial Appendage Occlusion Devices

David Begley*

Papworth Hospital, Cambridge

Abstract: Atrial fibrillation is the commonest sustained arrhythmia and is the commonest cause of stroke due to embolization of thrombi from the left atrium. Risk of stroke increases with age and other co-morbidities and can be reduced by oral anticoagulation with warfarin. However warfarin has a narrow therapeutic window and can be affected by drugs and some foods, resulting in many patients being inadequately anti-coagulated. In addition other patients may have contra-indications to its use. Surgical and echocardiographic studies have demonstrated the source of thrombi to be the left atrial appendage in over 90% of cases. Therefore excluding the left atrial appendage from the systemic circulation may be a viable alternative to anti-coagulation in reducing the risk of stroke.

Three devices have been developed for percutaneous deployment to exclude the left atrial appendage. The Percutaneous Left Atrial Appendage Transcatheter Occlusion System - PLAATO (ev3), Watchman (Aritech) and Amplatzer Cardiac Plug (AGA Medical) are all delivered *via* the femoral vein with transpetal access to the left atrium. Each consists of a self-expanding nitinol mesh which is lodged in the left atrial appendage occluding the appendage and allowing endothelialisation of the atrial facing surface.

Early non-randomized studies demonstrated the technique to be simple and feasible with acceptable risks associated with implantation. A recent randomized controlled trial comparing device occlusion of the appendage to warfarin demonstrated that the device was at least non-inferior to warfarin in preventing stroke in non-valvular atrial fibrillation.

ATRIAL FIBRILLATION, STROKE AND ORAL ANTICOAGULATION

Atrial fibrillation is the commonest sustained cardiac arrhythmia characterized by disorganised atrial activation resulting in ineffective and inefficient atrial contraction.[1] Atrial fibrillation becomes more prevalent with advancing age and as such, the incidence is likely to increase in line with an aging population, [1-5] and the overall lifetime risk of developing atrial fibrillation is one in four for subjects over the age of 40 [6].

One of the most serious and debilitating complications of atrial fibrillation is stroke as a consequence of embolization of left atrial thrombus. Atrial fibrillation is responsible for over 15% of all strokes [7]. The rate of stroke in various subgroups of patients with atrial fibrillation ranges from 2-10% per year increasing with age and other co-morbidities including history of hypertension, diabetes mellitus, previous cerebro-vascular event and recent congestive cardiac failure [8]. Stratification of risk allows selection of patients for oral anticoagulation, thereby minimizing the risk without exposing patients unnecessarily to an increased risk of bleeding [8, 9].

Randomised controlled trials have shown that anticoagulation with warfarin is effective in reducing the risk of stroke with a relative risk reduction of 62% compared to 22% with aspirin [10,11]. This would indicate that those patients at high risk of stroke should receive warfarin. Where the risk of stroke is low, bleeding complications from anticoagulation with warfarin may outweigh the benefits and therefore patients may be better managed with aspirin [12,13]. Antiarrhythmic drugs and more recently catheter ablation have proven effective in improving symptoms in patients with atrial fibrillation but are insufficiently reliable in preventing thromboembolic complications [14-18]. Therefore there is often a continuing need for long-term oral anticoagulation.

Despite the proven benefits of warfarin in preventing thromboembolic complications in atrial fibrillation it may be poorly tolerated by patients and has a narrow therapeutic range requiring frequent monitoring and dose adjustments [19]. In addition numerous medications and some foods interact adversely resulting in a level of anticoagulation outside this therapeutic range. As a result as many as 50% of patients who would benefit from long-term anticoagulation remain untreated [20]. Although numerous alternatives to warfarin are in development that may resolve some of these issues and prove as effective as warfarin, they will not address the primary problem of bleeding complications [21,22].

*Address correspondence to David Begley:** Papworth Hospital. Cambridge, UK; E-mail: David.Begley@papworth.nhs.uk

Peter M. Schofield (Ed)

Echocardiography and autopsy studies have demonstrated that the source of thrombi in non-valvular atrial fibrillation is the left atrial appendage in over 90% of cases[23, 24] and therefore strategies aimed at excluding the left atrial appendage from the systemic circulation may be a viable alternative to chronic anticoagulation in selected patients who would otherwise benefit from warfarin therapy [25].

DEVICE CLOSURE OF THE LEFT ATRIAL APPENDAGE

PLAATO (Percutaneous Left Atrial Appendage Transcatheter Occlusion) System (ev3 Inc., Plymouth, Minnesota)

The PLAATO device is a nitinol self-expanding framework with an expandable polytetrafluoroethylene (ePTFE) cover designed to lodge in the left atrial appendage to allow complete thrombosis within the device and later benign endothelialisation on the surface facing the left atrium.

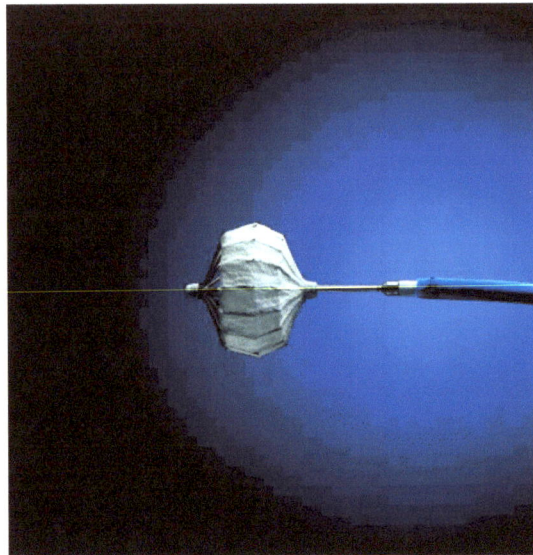

The device is introduced *via* the femoral vein with transeptal access to the left atrium. The device is positioned accurately within the left atrial appendage with fluoroscopic and transesophageal echo guidance. Once in position the device is expanded before removal of the delivery device.

A initial feasibility study was performed in 25 dogs [26]. Follow-up was performed between 2 days and 6 months after implantation. After follow-up dogs were euthanized and the left atrial appendage excised for examination. All left atrial appendages were occluded with no mobile thrombi seen. Healing on the atrial surface was complete by 3 months. Further examination of brain, kidney and spleen revealed no emboli or infarction.

Subsequently several human feasibility studies were performed [27-31]. In two of these studies devices were successfully implanted in 108 of 111 patients (97.3%) One patient had 2 major adverse events within the first 30 days: need for cardiac surgery and subsequent neurological death. Three other patients required surgery for hemopericardium. During a mean follow-up of 9.8 months 2 patients had a stroke. However there was no device migration or mobile thrombus observed on transesophageal echocardiography.

Three year follow-up in 11 patients reported a 3% annual stroke risk in a population with a predicted stroke risk of 8.6% per year [32]. They concluded that the device resulted in a stroke risk comparable to patients taking warfarin. There were no long-term complications related to the device.

More recently 5 year follow-up results of patients enrolled in the North American feasibility study have been published [33]. Patients were risk stratified before enrolment using the CHADS$_2$ scoring system. Study patients had an expected annual stroke/TIA risk of 6.6% per year with the actual stroke/TIA rate being 3.8% per year after 5 years follow-up – a 42% reduction. During follow-up there were 7 deaths, 5 major strokes, 3 minor strokes, 1 cardiac tamponade, 1 cerebral haemorrhage and 1 myocardial infarction. Only the cardiac tamponade was thought related to the device implantation.

The PLAATO device was withdrawn in 2006 before a definitive phase II study was performed with the company citing commercial reasons. There are currently no plans for a randomized trial using this device.

Watchman Left Atrial Appendage System (Aritech, Plymouth, Minnesota)

The Watchman left atrial appendage system is also constructed of nitinol. The atrial-facing surface is covered in a permeable polyester material. It is delivered *via* a catheter to the left atrial appendage with fluoroscopic and transesophageal echo guidance.

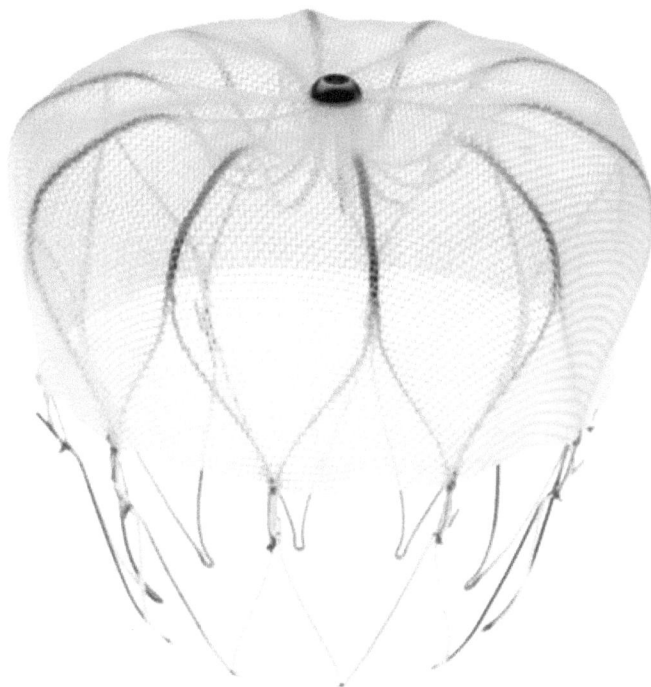

The PROTECT AF (WATCHMAN Left Atrial Appendage System for Embolic Protection in Patients with Atrial Fibrillation) study [34] was a multi-centre prospective, randomized controlled trial investigating the efficacy and safety of left atrial appendage occlusion in patients with non-valvular atrial fibrillation. It was designed to assess non-inferiority compared to chronic warfarin therapy. Patients over 18 years of age with paroxysmal or persistent atrial fibrillation with a CHADS [2] score of 1 or greater.

Seven hundred and seven eligible patients were enrolled. 463 were randomized to receive device closure of the left atrial appendage and 244 received warfarin treatment. Efficacy was determined by a primary end-point of stroke, cardiovascular death, or systemic embolization.

The primary efficacy event rate in the treatment group was 3.0 per 100 patient years compared to 4.9 per 100 patient years in the control group. The probability of non-inferiority in the intervention group was greater than 99.9%. Serious adverse events were more frequent in the treatment group compared to the control group. (7.4 per 100 patient years *vs* 4.4 per 100 patient years).

Amplatzer Cardiac Plug (AGA Medical, Plymouth, Minnesota)

The Amplatzer Cardiac Plug is a self expanding nitinol mesh consisting of a lobe designed to conform to the inner wall of the left atrial appendage. The lobe is connected by an articulating, compliant waist to a disc which is intended to sit flush to the atrial wall under slight tension and completely occlude the orifice.

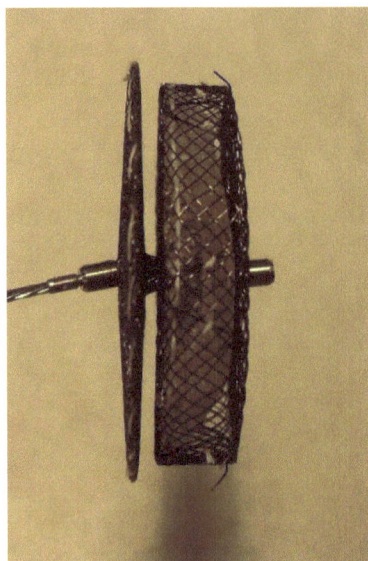

The Cardiac Plug was developed from the Amplatzer Septal Occluder, a device initially intended for closure of atrial septal defects. There is less clinical experience with the Amplatzer device compared to the Watchman device but does offer some potential advantages relating to the nature of the disc which creates a flush occlusion of the appendage.

SUMMARY

The prevalence of atrial fibrillation is increasing in parallel to an aging population and is the commonest cause of stroke. Anticoagulation is effective in reducing the stroke rate in high risk patients but may be unsuitable in as many as 50% of patients who would benefit. The left atrial appendage is the most frequent source of thrombi in non-valvular atrial fibrillation. Percutaneous occlusion of the left atrial appendage has been proven a simple and feasible technique. Additional evidence has shown it to be at least as efficacious as warfarin therapy in high risk patients. However there is a slightly higher risk of serious adverse events relating to device implantation. Further evidence is still needed on long-term efficacy and safety.

REFERENCES

[1] Miyasaka Y, Barnes ME, Gersh BJ, *et al*. Secular trends in incidence of atrial fibrillation in Olmsted County, Minnesota, 1980 to 2000, and implications on the projections for future prevalence. Circulation 2006 July 11; 114(2): 119-25.

[2] Benjamin EJ, Levy D, Vaziri SM, D'Agostino RB, Belanger AJ, Wolf PA. Independent risk factors for atrial fibrillation in a population-based cohort. The Framingham Heart Study. JAMA 1994 March 16; 271(11): 840-4.

[3] Psaty BM, Manolio TA, Kuller LH, *et al*. Incidence of and risk factors for atrial fibrillation in older adults. Circulation 1997 October 7; 96(7): 2455-61.

[4] Ruigomez A, Johansson S, Wallander MA, Rodriguez LA. Incidence of chronic atrial fibrillation in general practice and its treatment pattern. J Clin Epidemiol 2002 April; 55(4): 358-63.

[5] Stewart S, Hart CL, Hole DJ, McMurray JJ. Population prevalence, incidence, and predictors of atrial fibrillation in the Renfrew/Paisley study. Heart 2001 November; 86(5): 516-21.

[6] Lloyd-Jones DM, Wang TJ, Leip EP, *et al*. Lifetime risk for development of atrial fibrillation: the Framingham Heart Study. Circulation 2004 August 31; 110(9): 1042-6.

[7] Sandercock P, Bamford J, Dennis M, *et al*. Atrial fibrillation and stroke: prevalence in different types of stroke and influence on early and long term prognosis (Oxfordshire community stroke project). BMJ 1992 December 12; 305(6867): 1460-5.

[8] Gage BF, Waterman AD, Shannon W, Boechler M, Rich MW, Radford MJ. Validation of clinical classification schemes for predicting stroke: results from the National Registry of Atrial Fibrillation. JAMA 2001 June 13; 285(22): 2864-70.

[9] Gage BF, van WC, Pearce L, *et al*. Selecting patients with atrial fibrillation for anticoagulation: stroke risk stratification in patients taking aspirin. Circulation 2004 October 19; 110(16): 2287-92.

[10]   Hart RG, Benavente O, McBride R, Pearce LA. Antithrombotic therapy to prevent stroke in patients with atrial fibrillation: a meta-analysis. Ann Intern Med 1999 October 5; 131(7): 492-501.

[11]   Risk factors for stroke and efficacy of antithrombotic therapy in atrial fibrillation. Analysis of pooled data from five randomized controlled trials. Arch Intern Med 1994 July 11; 154(13): 1449-57.

[12]   Gage BF, Cardinalli AB, Albers GW, Owens DK. Cost-effectiveness of warfarin and aspirin for prophylaxis of stroke in patients with nonvalvular atrial fibrillation. JAMA 1995 December 20; 274(23): 1839-45.

[13]   Laupacis A, Albers G, Dalen J, Dunn MI, Jacobson AK, Singer DE. Antithrombotic therapy in atrial fibrillation. Chest 1998 November; 114(5 Suppl): 579S-89S.

[14]   Levitt HL, Toor SZ, Coplan NL. Is there a need to continue anticoagulation following "successful" atrial fibrillation ablation? Prev Cardiol 2009; 12(1): 39-42.

[15]   Sherman DG, Kim SG, Boop BS, *et al.* Occurrence and characteristics of stroke events in the Atrial Fibrillation Follow-up Investigation of Sinus Rhythm Management (AFFIRM) study. Arch Intern Med 2005 May 23; 165(10): 1185-91.

[16]   Sherman DG. Stroke prevention in atrial fibrillation: pharmacological rate versus rhythm control. Stroke 2007 February; 38(2 Suppl): 615-7.

[17]   Van Gelder IC, Hagens VE, Bosker HA, *et al.* A comparison of rate control and rhythm control in patients with recurrent persistent atrial fibrillation. N Engl J Med 2002 December 5; 347(23): 1834-40.

[18]   Wyse DG, Waldo AL, Dimarco JP, *et al.* A comparison of rate control and rhythm control in patients with atrial fibrillation. N Engl J Med 2002 December 5; 347(23): 1825-33.

[19]   Walker AM, Bennett D. Epidemiology and outcomes in patients with atrial fibrillation in the United States. Heart Rhythm 2008 October; 5(10): 1365-72.

[20]   Go AS, Hylek EM, Borowsky LH, Phillips KA, Selby JV, Singer DE. Warfarin use among ambulatory patients with nonvalvular atrial fibrillation: the anticoagulation and risk factors in atrial fibrillation (ATRIA) study. Ann Intern Med 1999 December 21; 131(12): 927-34.

[21]   Albers GW, Diener HC, Frison L, *et al.* Ximelagatran vs warfarin for stroke prevention in patients with nonvalvular atrial fibrillation: a randomized trial. JAMA 2005 February 9; 293(6): 690-8.

[22]   Connolly S, Pogue J, Hart R, *et al.* Clopidogrel plus aspirin versus oral anticoagulation for atrial fibrillation in the Atrial fibrillation Clopidogrel Trial with Irbesartan for prevention of Vascular Events (ACTIVE W): a randomised controlled trial. Lancet 2006 June 10; 367(9526): 1903-12.

[23]   Blackshear JL, Odell JA. Appendage obliteration to reduce stroke in cardiac surgical patients with atrial fibrillation. Ann Thorac Surg 1996 February; 61(2): 755-9.

[24]   Stoddard MF, Dawkins PR, Prince CR, Ammash NM. Left atrial appendage thrombus is not uncommon in patients with acute atrial fibrillation and a recent embolic event: a transesophageal echocardiographic study. J Am Coll Cardiol 1995 February; 25(2): 452-9.

[25]   Garcia-Fernandez MA, Perez-David E, Quiles J, *et al.* Role of left atrial appendage obliteration in stroke reduction in patients with mitral valve prosthesis: a transesophageal echocardiographic study. J Am Coll Cardiol 2003 October 1; 42(7): 1253-8.

[26]   Nakai T, Lesh MD, Gerstenfeld EP, Virmani R, Jones R, Lee RJ. Percutaneous left atrial appendage occlusion (PLAATO) for preventing cardioembolism: first experience in canine model. Circulation 2002 May 7; 105(18): 2217-22.

[27]   Himbert D, Cachier A, Brochet E, *et al.* [Feasibility of percutaneous exclusion of the left atrial appendage: results of 11 cases]. Arch Mal Coeur Vaiss 2006 June; 99(6): 585-92.

[28]   Ussia GP, Mangiafico S, Privitera A, *et al.* Percutaneous left atrial appendage transcatheter occlusion in patients with chronic nonvalvular atrial fibrillation: early institutional experience. J Cardiovasc Med (Hagerstown) 2006 August; 7(8): 569-72.

[29]   Ostermayer SH, Reisman M, Kramer PH, *et al.* Percutaneous left atrial appendage transcatheter occlusion (PLAATO system) to prevent stroke in high-risk patients with non-rheumatic atrial fibrillation: results from the international multi-center feasibility trials. J Am Coll Cardiol 2005 July 5; 46(1): 9-14.

[30]   Omran H, Hardung D, Schmidt H, Hammerstingl C, Luderitz B. Mechanical occlusion of the left atrial appendage. J Cardiovasc Electrophysiol 2003 September; 14(9 Suppl): S56-S59.

[31]   Sievert H, Lesh MD, Trepels T, *et al.* Percutaneous left atrial appendage transcatheter occlusion to prevent stroke in high-risk patients with atrial fibrillation: early clinical experience. Circulation 2002 April 23; 105(16): 1887-9.

[32]   El-Chami MF, Grow P, Eilen D, Lerakis S, Block PC. Clinical outcomes three years after PLAATO implantation. Catheter Cardiovasc Interv 2007 April 1; 69(5): 704-7.

[33]   Block PC, Burstein S, Casale PN, *et al.* Percutaneous left atrial appendage occlusion for patients in atrial fibrillation suboptimal for warfarin therapy: 5-year results of the PLAATO (Percutaneous Left Atrial Appendage Transcatheter Occlusion) Study. JACC Cardiovasc Interv 2009 July; 2(7): 594-600.

[34] Holmes DR, Reddy VY, Turi ZG, *et al.* Percutaneous closure of the left atrial appendage versus warfarin therapy for prevention of stroke in patients with atrial fibrillation: a randomised non-inferiority trial. Lancet 2009 August 15; 374(9689): 534-42.

Index

A

Amplatzer cardiac plug 110–111
Amplatzer device 14, 19
Aortic stenosis 21-23, 56-61
Aortic valvuloplasty 61-63
Atrial fibrillation 108-109
Atrial septal defect
- Anatomy 18
- Closure 18-19
- Complications of closure 20
- Imaging 18

B

BioSTAR device 14, 19

C

CARILLON device 101, 103-104
Corevalve 26

E

Edwards Sapien valve 25-26

H

HELEX device 14, 19

I

Inoue technique 69-74
- Complications 74
- Results 75

M

Mitraclip device 95-98
Mitral stenosis 63-66
Mitral valve
- Anatomy 90-92
- Regurgitation 92-94, 99-101
Mitral valvuloplasty 66-69
Mitralign device 104-105
MONARC device 101, 103

P

Patent foramen ovale
- Anatomy 3
- Complications 4-5, 15-16
- Epidemiology 3-4
- Imaging 5-10
- Treatment 11-15

www.ingramcontent.com/pod-product-compliance
Lightning Source LLC
Chambersburg PA
CBHW041718210326
41598CB00007B/698